D0553029

Hatha Yoga
· Manual I ·

Hatha Yoga
· Manual I ·

by
Saṁskṛti and Veda

Second Edition,
Revised and Expanded

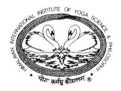

The Himalayan International Institute
of Yoga Science and Philosophy of the U.S.A.
Honesdale, Pennsylvania

©1977 and 1985 by The Himalayan International Institute
of Yoga Science and Philosophy of the U.S.A.
RR 1, Box 400
Honesdale, Pennsylvania 18431

All rights reserved. No part of this book may be reproduced in any form or by any means without
permission in writing from the publisher. Printed in the United States of America.

The paper used in this publication meets the minimum requirements of American National Standard for
Information Sciences—Permanence of Paper for Printed Library Materials, ANSI Z39.48–1984.
∞

Library of Congress Cataloging in Publication Data:

Saṁskṛti.
    Hatha yoga.

    Includes index.
    1. Yoga, Hatha. I. Veda. II. Title.
RA781.7.S25   1986   613.7′046   86-4757
ISBN 0-89389-082-0

Dedicated to our
reverend teacher Shri Swami Rama of the Himalayas,
from whom we have been learning.

Special thanks are due to Wendy Hoffman and Barb Bova, who spent innumerable hours working on the revised edition of this manual and organizing it in a manner consistent with the classes taught by the Himalayan Institute Teachers' Association. Without their help and encouragement this edition would not have come into being.

The authors would also like to express thanks to the following people, whose work was invaluable in bringing this book to print: Shri O. P. Tiwari, David Coulter, Ph.D., Dave Gorman, Ron Glick, and Shirley Walter.

ॐ सह नाववतु। सह नौ भुनक्तु।
सह वीर्यं करवावहै। तेजस्वि नाव
धीतमस्तु। मा विद्विषावहै।
ॐ शान्तिः। शान्तिः।। शान्तिः।।।

Prayer of Harmony

for Teacher and Student

OM saha na vavatu
saha nau bhunaktu
saha viryam karavavahai
tejasvi navadhitamastu
ma vidvishavahai
OM shantih shantih shantih

O God, protect us both together,
Accept us both together,
Let us achieve strength,
Let our learning ever shine,
Let us not resent each other.
OM Peace Peace Peace

Contents

Introduction by Pandit Rajmani Tigunait, Ph.D.   1

How to Use This Manual   3

Attitudes, Hints, and Cautions   6

Yamas and Niyamas   8

Diaphragmatic Breathing   10

Relaxation Postures   13

    Corpse (*Shavasana*)   14
    Crocodile (*Makarasana*)   16
    Child's Posture (*Balasana*)   18
    Knees-to-Chest Posture   20
    Simple Standing Posture   21

Stretching and Limbering Exercises   23

    Symmetrical Stretch   24
    Cat Stretch   26
    Horizontal Stretch   28
    Overhead Stretch   30
    Side Stretch   32
    Simple Back Stretch   34
    Torso Twist   36
    Swimming Stretch   38
    Churning (*Chalan*)   40

Sun Salutation (*Surya Namaskara*)   43

Asanas and Preparatory Exercises   61

    A. Standing Postures   65

    Abdominal Lift (*Uddiyana Bandha*)   66
    Angle Posture (*Konasana*)   68
    Triangle (*Trikonasana*)   72
    Preparation for Revolving Triangle   74
    Revolving Triangle (*Parivritta Trikonasana*)   76
    Tree (*Vrikshasana*)   78
    Preparation for Hand-to-Foot Posture   82
    Hand-to-Foot Posture (*Padahastasana*)   84

    B. Sitting Postures   87

    Easy Posture (*Sukhasana*)   88

Kneeling Posture (*Vajrasana*)   89
Half Lotus (*Ardha Padmasana*)   90
Leg Cradles   92
Butterfly   96
Lion (*Simhasana*)   98
Symbol of Yoga (*Yoga Mudra*)   100
Squatting Posture   102
Cow's Face (*Gomukhasana*)   104

C. Backward-Bending Postures   109

Cobra (*Bhujangasana*)   110
Horse Mudra (*Ashvini Mudra*)   112
Half Boat (*Ardha Naukasana*)   114
Boat (*Naukasana*)   116
Half Locust (*Ardha Shalabhasana*)   118
Locust (*Shalabhasana*)   119
Half Bow (*Ardha Dhanurasana*)   120
Bow (*Dhanurasana*)   122

D. Forward-Bending Postures   124

Preparation for Head-to-Knee Posture and Posterior Stretch   125
Head-to-Knee Posture (*Janushirshasana*)   126
Posterior Stretch (*Paschimottanasana*)   128
Inclined Plane (*Katikasana*)   130

E. Twisting Postures   133

Twisting Posture   134
Half Spinal Twist (*Ardha Matsyendrasana*)   136

F. Leg Lifts   138

Wind-Eliminating Posture (*Pavanamuktasana*)   139
Single Leg Lifts (*Utthita Ekapadasana*)   140
Double Leg Lifts (*Utthita Dvipadasana*)   143
Balance on Hips (*Utthita Hastapadasana*)   144

G. Inverted Postures   147

Rocking Chair   148
Half Plow (*Ardha Halasana*)   150
Plow (*Halasana*)   152
Inverted Action Posture (*Vipritakarani*)   154
Shoulderstand (*Sarvangasana*)   156
Arch Posture   158
Half Fish (*Ardha Matsyasana*)   159
Preparation for the Headstand   160
Headstand (*Shirshasana*)   162

Relaxation Exercises   167

Tension/Relaxation Exercise   168
Complete Relaxation Exercise   169

Breathing Exercises   171

     The Complete Breath   173
     Nadi Shodhana   173
     Kapalabhati Pranayama   174

Appendix A: Sample Lesson Plans   175

Appendix B: Hatha Yoga and Menstruation—by Barbara Bova   182

About the Authors   184

The Himalayan Institute Teachers' Association and Diploma Program   185

Index   186

Introduction

Yoga is one of the six schools of Indian philosophy. Unlike the other schools, it is accepted not only as a philosophy but also as a science and a practical method of self-unfoldment, the application of which can lead to the absolute Truth. Because of this emphasis on practice rather than theory, the other schools of philosophy frequently refer to and utilize the experiences of the yogis, particularly their exploration of the conscious, unconscious, and superconscious levels of their being.

In the history of Indian philosophy, yoga developed in many different aspects, including karma yoga, the yoga of action; bhakti yoga, the yoga of devotion; and jnana yoga, the yoga of knowledge. Besides the development of these different methods of spiritual practice, hatha yoga gained popularity among ascetics and those interested in the physiological conditions of the body and the control of breath. Because of its emphasis on *asanas* (postures) and *pranayama* (breath control) rather than on philosophical matters, hatha yoga was not accepted as a formal school of philosophy.

Raja yoga, the royal path—which is correctly called ashtanga yoga, the eightfold path—includes the teachings of all paths of yoga. The practice and philosophy of raja yoga was codified by Patanjali, approximately A.D. 200, in his Yoga Sutras, a work consisting of 196 aphorisms or sutras. The eight *angas*—limbs or rungs—of this path are:

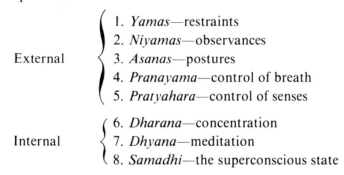

External
1. *Yamas*—restraints
2. *Niyamas*—observances
3. *Asanas*—postures
4. *Pranayama*—control of breath
5. *Pratyahara*—control of senses

Internal
6. *Dharana*—concentration
7. *Dhyana*—meditation
8. *Samadhi*—the superconscious state

Patanjali describes the *yamas, niyamas, asanas, pranayama,* and *pratyahara* as external forms of practice and *dharana, dhyana,* and *samadhi* as internal forms.

Patanjali's teaching of raja yoga begins with the five *yamas* and the five *niyamas,* the moral disciplines of yoga. These disciplines are as important for the beginning student as they are for the accomplished yogi.

In his Yoga Sutras, Patanjali accepts some principles of hatha yoga, but does not describe *asanas* or *pranayama* in detail. He emphasizes concentration (*dharana*) and meditation (*dhyana*).

In chapter 2, sutra 46, Patanjali defines *asana* as "a particular posture of the body, which is steady and comfortable." In the system of raja yoga this definition applies to those postures that are used in the practice of meditation. This is made clear in sutra 47: "The posture is perfected, made steady and comfortable, through relaxing, not forcing the effort, and by fixing the consciousness on the Infinite."

The hatha yoga school treats the subject of asanas, pranayama, and other more subtle forms of practice at great length. Its exponents developed these aspects of raja yoga after Patanjali's codification of the Yoga Sutras. Sometime around the fifteenth century Svatmarama systematized and codified the science of hatha yoga in his extensive work, the *Hathayogapradipika.*

In this classical text on hatha yoga, Svatmarama explains that "ha" represents the sun and "tha" represents the moon. Hatha yoga thus means the practice of uniting the sun and the moon. "Ha" and "tha" are also symbolic expressions of *pingala* and *ida* (the two main channels of subtle energy in the body), of *prana* and *apana* (the upward-flowing energy and the downward-flowing energy), of right and left, of male and female, of active and passive.

Svatmarama begins the *Hathayogapradipika* by explaining that hatha yoga is a stairway for those who wish to attain the heights of raja yoga. Thus, yoga should not be practiced for the sake of perfecting the postures only. This is a particular problem in the West, where yoga has become especially popular in the form of hatha yoga. The goal of hatha yoga ultimately is to attain the goal of raja yoga, that is, Self-realization.

There are at least eighty-four basic *asanas*, with numerous variations. It is not always easy to discover which postures should be practiced by beginning students and which should be practiced by advanced students. In this book, the writers have included those asanas that are easy and beneficial for beginning students and have paid particular attention to the needs and abilities of Western students. If students follow the practices of this book as outlined they will be greatly aided in understanding the basic principles of hatha yoga.

Pandit Rajmani Tigunait, Ph.D.

How to Use This Manual

This manual is designed for students who have had no exposure to hatha yoga or who have recently begun to practice. Read the sections "Attitudes, Hints, and Cautions," "Yamas and Niyamas," and "Diaphragmatic Breathing" carefully before attempting any of the exercises or postures. Many of the postures have been simplified, but in such a way that the benefits have not been minimized. The preliminary steps shown are important in order to perfect the postures; master them before adding the advanced variations. If you have no serious physical problems, you can successfully learn most of the postures in three to four months of daily practice. It is important to read all the instructions, including the preliminary exercises, cautions, and benefits, before attempting a posture. Remember that no manual on a practical subject, such as hatha yoga, can substitute for studying with a qualified teacher. If you are practicing on your own, exercise care and common sense at all times.

We recommend two supplementary texts in conjunction with this manual: *Joints and Glands Exercises,* edited by Rudolph M. Ballentine, M.D., and *Lectures on Yoga,* by Swami Rama. Both are published by the Himalayan Institute. The joints and glands exercises and the stretching exercises should be practiced for two to three weeks before beginning the postures. Older persons as well as those who have not performed physical exercise for some time should practice these exercises for a longer period. *Lectures on Yoga* gives a philosophical overview of the eight-runged system of raja yoga and discusses the yamas (the first rung), niyamas (the second rung), and pranayama (the fourth rung) in greater detail than we do here in this manual. Our main focus in this manual is of course on asanas (the third rung).

After reading the section on diaphragmatic breathing, spend a few minutes each day practicing diaphragmatic breathing until it becomes a natural function. In all the exercises and asanas, deep, even breathing is recommended. Beginners should not practice breath retention in any of the postures.

Every day practice a few stretching exercises, as well as the sun salutation, in order to limber the body before beginning the asanas. If preparatory exercises are shown for an asana, practice them for one to two weeks before attempting the asana itself.

If you have recently undergone surgery, or have any serious physical problem, or have glaucoma or a tendency toward high blood pressure, check with your physician before beginning the practice of hatha yoga. People with either glaucoma or a tendency toward high blood pressure are especially warned against attempting any inverted posture without the approval of their physician.

Begin with three repetitions of each posture. Slowly increase the duration of each posture and reduce the repetitions.

Balance is an important principle of hatha yoga. Backward-bending postures should be balanced with forward-bending postures. You can follow a forward bend with a backward bend (such as in the second and third positions of the sun salutation), or a number of backward-bending asanas with a number of forward-bending asanas. This basic principle of balance also applies to the repetitions of asanas. If you practice an exercise or asana three times on one side, practice it three times on the opposite side. However, if one side of the body is more stiff than the other, practice extra repetitions on that side until both are equally supple.

Students should begin with the standing postures and end with the headstand. But other than that there are no hard and fast rules about the sequence of practicing postures. For the sake of clarity the postures in this manual are presented in an order that is a good general guide for practice, working from the active warm-up exercises to those postures that move the body less. The basic sequence used is

stretching and limbering exercises
standing postures
sitting and meditative postures
backward-bending postures
forward-bending postures
twisting postures
leg lifts
inverted postures
relaxation
breathing exercises

In addition to the general limbering exercises done at the beginning of the sequence to prepare the body for doing the postures, other stretching and limbering exercises are included within the different categories. These focus on increasing flexibility and agility of specific areas or parts of the body and are often listed as preparatory exercises for a particular posture. For example, the rocking chair, which may be used as a general limbering exercise, has been put with the inverted postures because it is practiced as a preparation for the half plow. You may find it helpful to practice these stretching and preparatory exercises for some time if you experience difficulty doing the actual postures.

Begin with the abdominal lift, the stretching and limbering exercises, the sun salutation, and the standing postures. The backward-bending postures slowly and gently limber the spinal column for the more difficult asanas. In the backward-bending postures there are two important points to remain aware of: the neck and the small of the back. The backward-bending postures are counterbalanced with the forward-bending postures. The fish should always follow the shoulderstand and plow, as it counterbalances the extreme forward bend in the neck from these two postures. Read with extra care the cautions and hints for the headstand before attempting the posture.

Relax in the postures, be aware of the breath, and concentrate on the area of stretch. Move smoothly and gently going into, holding, and coming out of the postures. By keeping the breath even, smooth, and deep, each posture can be held with little or no movement. This is the first step in perfecting the asanas and in preparing to sit in a steady and comfortable posture for meditation.

Relaxation between asanas can be done in either the crocodile posture, the child's posture, or the corpse posture. The crocodile is used to relax between the postures done lying on the stomach, the child's pose after a series of backward-bending postures, and the corpse before and after the entire sequence of postures, and also between the postures lying on the back.

If you experience difficulty doing a posture, first mentally envision yourself doing it, *then* do it physically. If you can't do it mentally, *don't* do it physically.

All the postures described in this manual with the exception of the easy posture, *sukhasana,* and the kneeling posture, *vajrasana,* are cultural postures, that is, they are asanas for physical well-being. In this manual the kneeling posture has been used only as a preparation for a few of the cultural postures, and the half lotus as a preparation for the full lotus posture. A presentation of the various meditative asanas can be found in *Hatha Yoga Manual II* by Saṁskṛti and Judith Franks, a Himalayan Institute publication.

Practice the channel purification exercise (*nadi shodhana*) after the asanas and the complete relaxation exercise.

If there are times when you are unable to practice all the postures, then choose one or two of each type. Be certain to include the abdominal lift, some stretching and limbering exercises, the sun salutation, the cobra, a forward-bending posture, a twisting posture, the plow-shoulderstand-fish series, and a balance posture. Appendix A of this manual provides sample 30-minute, 60-minute, and 90-minute lesson plans for both the beginning I and beginning II levels of practice.

Attitudes, Hints, and Cautions

Asanas, unlike other physical disciplines, are not correctly practiced unless the proper mental attitudes are cultivated; they should be practiced with patience, determination, and joy. A number of preparations are helpful in bringing about the proper mood.

• Set a specific time each day for your practice. This should be a time when you do not feel pressured into rushing through the postures. Pick a time when the likelihood of disturbances is at a minimum. It is also important to practice your postures every day, regularly. In this way you will find yourself unconsciously preparing for the postures before actually beginning them.

• The most beneficial times to practice asanas are the mornings and evenings. Practicing asanas in the morning helps you remain calm and alert the entire day. In the evening, asanas relieve the day's tensions and help you to later enjoy an undisturbed and peaceful sleep. In the morning the body is stiffer, so take greater care practicing your asanas. A warm bath or shower when you first get up will help relax your muscles. Then, before beginning the asanas, practice sufficient stretching and limbering exercises. You should save the more difficult asanas for the evening.

• Practice your asanas in a clean, quiet, well-ventilated area that is free from drafts. Wear loose and comfortable clothing; cotton or other natural materials are best, for they allow the body to breathe. It may also be helpful to have an "asana suit" or set of clothing that you use exclusively for your practice.

• Always practice postures on an empty stomach. Wait at least four hours after a heavy meal and two hours after a light meal. Do not drink liquids immediately before doing postures. As we state in the introduction to the asanas, many of the postures increase intra-abdominal pressure and affect the internal organs. Practicing with food in the stomach will cause discomfort and can lead to more serious problems. For this same reason we also recommend that the bowels and bladder be empty.

• Women should not practice asanas during menstruation. (See Appendix B, p. 182.) This is a natural cleansing time in which many physical and physiological changes occur, so you should allow your body to rest. Practicing asanas during menstruation may cause cramps and excessive bleeding. Also, during pregnancy you should check with your physician before continuing any of the exercises or asanas.

• Do not become discouraged if your body does not respond in the same way each day. Sometimes you will discover that the posture you found easy yesterday is not so easy today. It takes time and regular practice for both the body and mind to stabilize. The important thing is to keep practicing regularly. Approach each day's practice as an opportunity to study anew the body's movements and capacities.

Never develop a sense of competition either with fellow students or with yourself. This reduces your practice of asanas to a level of mere physical performance.

• Study your body and its movements. Be aware of your capacity and learn not to go beyond it. In any posture, concentrate the mind on the muscles that are being stretched and learn to distinguish between stretching and straining. Any shaking, straining, or pain indicates either that you are doing something incorrectly or that you have gone beyond your capacity. Gentleness and regularity in practice is far superior to forcing the body into a posture prematurely. Let common sense prevail.

• Let the body movements flow evenly and gently with the breath. Generally, whenever you expand the chest you will inhale naturally; whenever you bend the torso toward the lower half of the body you will exhale. Breathe evenly and deeply without jerks and pauses. The breath, however, should not become a source of distraction through overconscientiousness; it should be allowed to flow easily and naturally. In almost all the postures, we have recommended even, deep breathing. Breath retention is not recommended for beginners.

• Follow any exertion by relaxation. The length of relaxation depends on each individual; your breathing and heartbeat should return to normal before doing the next posture. However, never allow the mind to drift toward sleep either between postures or during the relaxation exercise at the end of your postures.

Yamas and Niyamas

The *yamas* and *niyamas*, the first two rungs of ashtanga yoga, constitute the gateway through which we must pass if we are to enter the path of yoga. They are the moral foundation upon which the successful practice of yoga is built, and should be practiced to perfection on all levels—thought, word, and action. We are not, however, expected to master these principles completely before beginning the practice of asanas, pranayama, and the other rungs of yoga. The yamas and niyamas are ideals whose perfection we will become aware of on increasingly subtler levels as we progress on the path of yoga. It is necessary that the increased awareness and self-control obtained in the preliminary practice of yoga be used in a positive and constructive manner, as it is only those of pure mind and heart who can attain the highest states of their being.

The yamas are moral disciplines and restraints that regulate our relationships with other individuals. The niyamas are constructive observances designed to organize our personal daily lives. Briefly, the yamas and niyamas are as follows.

YAMAS

AHIMSA Nonviolence with mind, action, and speech; non-hurting, non-injuring, non-harming, and non-killing.

SATYA Truthfulness. This refers to the avoidance of all falsehood, exaggeration, and pretense, and is necessary for the unfoldment of our intuitive, discriminating faculties.

ASTEYA Non-stealing. This refers not only to stealing physical objects but also to taking credit for anything that is not rightly ours.

BRAHMACHARYA Literally, "walking in Brahman." The control of sensual desires, allowing us to use that energy for higher purposes. *Brahmacharya* is frequently translated as celibacy; however, it more properly refers to continence in either celibate or married life.

APARIGRAHA Non-possessiveness. This refers to using the things of the world for their intended purposes, without a feeling that we own them or that we are owned by them.

NIYAMAS

SHAUCHA Purity. We purify the body by eating pure, healthy foods and by practicing cleansing exercises. We purify the mind by ridding ourselves of undesirable thoughts and emotions.

SANTOSHA   Contentment. We should not allow outside influences to disturb our inner tranquility.

TAPAS   Literally, "that which generates heat." This refers to those actions, disciplines, and austerities that purify the mind and the body and increase our desire for enlightenment.

SVADHYAYA   Self-study. This refers to the study of the scriptures and of the internal states of consciousness.

ISHVARA PRANIDHANA   Literally, "surrender to the Ultimate." When we unite our individual will with that of a higher principle, all egotism, pettiness, and selfishness are removed.

Diaphragmatic Breathing

Although breathing is one of our most vital functions, it is little understood and often done improperly. Most people breathe shallowly and haphazardly, going against the natural rhythmic movement of the body's respiratory system. Diaphragmatic breathing, on the other hand, promotes a natural, even breath movement that strengthens the nervous system and relaxes the body. The importance of deep, even breathing in practicing the asanas cannot be overemphasized.

Respiration is normally of either of two types or a combination of both: costal or abdominal, according to Catherine P. Anthony in her *Textbook of Anatomy and Physiology* (St. Louis: C. V. Mosby Co., 1971, p. 376). Costal breathing (also called chest breathing or shallow breathing) is characterized by "an upward, outward movement of the chest due to contraction of the external intercostals and other chest-elevating muscles." Deep abdominal breathing is characterized by "an outward movement of the abdominal wall due to the contraction and descent of the diaphragm." Practitioners of yoga recognize a third type of breathing, known as diaphragmatic breathing, which focuses attention on the diaphragm in the lower rib cage. It is this method of breathing that is practiced during the asanas. Diaphragmatic breathing should not be confused with abdominal or belly breathing, which is also sometimes referred to as deep diaphragmatic breathing.

The principle muscle of diaphragmatic breathing, the diaphragm, is a strong, horizontal, dome-shaped muscle. It divides the thoracic cavity, which contains the heart and lungs, from the abdominal cavity, which contains the organs of digestion, reproduction, and excretion. The diaphragm is located approximately two finger-widths below the nipples in its relaxed or dome-shaped state. It comes up slightly higher on the right side (between the fourth and fifth ribs) than it does on the left side (between the fifth and sixth ribs). In the center the diaphragm is located at the xiphoid process, the lower part of the sterum. The rectus abdominis, the two strong vertical muscles of the abdomen, work in cooperation with the diaphragm during diaphragmatic breathing.

Location of the diaphragm in relation to the ribs and internal organs

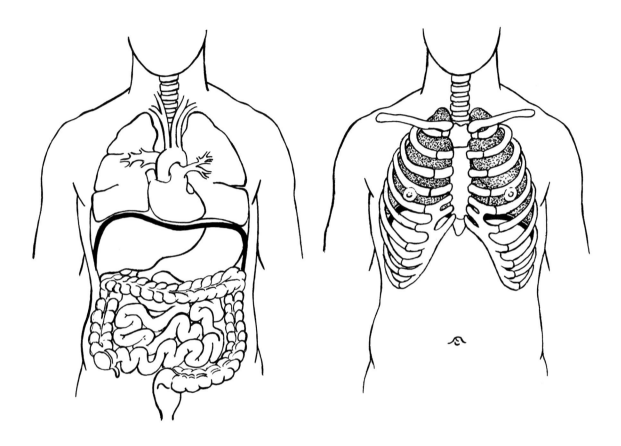

Drawings by Michael Smith

During inhalation the diaphragm contracts and flattens; it pushes downward, causing the upper abdominal muscles to relax and extend slightly and the lower "floating" ribs to flare slightly outward. In this position the lungs expand, creating a partial vacuum, which draws air into the chest cavity. During exhalation the diaphragm relaxes and returns to its dome-shaped position. During this upward movement the upper abdominal muscles contract, and carbon dioxide is forced from the lungs.

Movement during inhalation and exhalation

INHALATION   **EXHALATION**

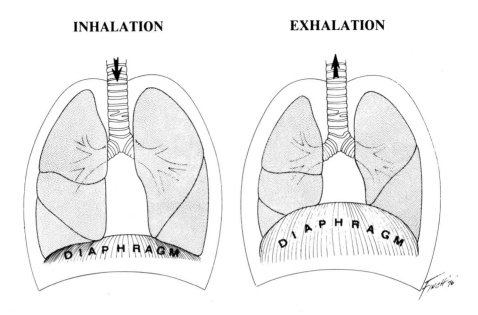

Diaphragmatic breathing has three important effects on the body:

1. In diaphragmatic breathing, unlike shallow breathing, the lungs fill completely, providing the body with sufficient oxygen.
2. Diaphragmatic breathing forces the waste product of the respiratory process, carbon dioxide, from the lungs. When breathing shallowly some carbon dioxide may remain trapped in the lungs, causing fatigue and nervousness.
3. The up and down motion of the diaphragm gently massages the abdominal organs; this increases circulation to these organs and thus aids in their functioning.

In diaphragmatic breathing a minimum amount of effort is used to receive a maximum amount of air; thus, it is our most efficient method of breathing.

Technique

Lie on the back with the feet a comfortable distance apart. Gently close the eyes and place one hand at the base of the rib cage and the other on the chest.

Inhale and exhale through the nostrils slowly, smoothly, and evenly, with no noise, jerks, or pauses in the breath. While inhaling, be aware of the upper abdominal muscles expanding and the lower ribs flaring out slightly. There should be little or no movement of the chest.

Practice this method of deep breathing 3 to 5 minutes daily until you clearly understand the movement of the diaphragm and the upper abdominal muscles. The body is designed to breathe diaphragmatically; gradually it should again become a natural function.

RELAXATION POSTURES

CORPSE (*Shavasana*)

Lie on the back and gently close the eyes. Place the feet a comfortable distance apart; place the arms away from the sides of the body, with the palms upward and the fingers gently curled. The legs should not touch each other, nor should the arms and hands touch the body. Do not lie haphazardly or place the limbs far apart, but lie in a symmetrical position, with the head, neck, and trunk aligned.

In this asana the body resembles a corpse; it lies still and relaxed. It is important to keep the mind alert and focused on the flow of the breath.

Between asanas, remain in this posture only until respiration and heartbeat return to normal. For relaxation before and after the entire sequence of asanas, beginners should not remain in this posture for more than ten minutes, in order to prevent drowsiness.

Beginning students can come out of the posture by raising the left arm overhead, rolling onto the left side, and gradually coming into a sitting position.

Benefits:

- Between postures, it helps you to relax and to prepare the mind for the next posture in the sequence.

- Before postures, it centers the mind and prepares it for focusing on the asanas. It helps you to relax the skeletal muscles, enabling you to go further into the postures while reducing the likelihood of injuries.

- After postures, it reduces fatigue.

- At midday, as a break from your work, it relaxes and rejuvenates the mind and body.

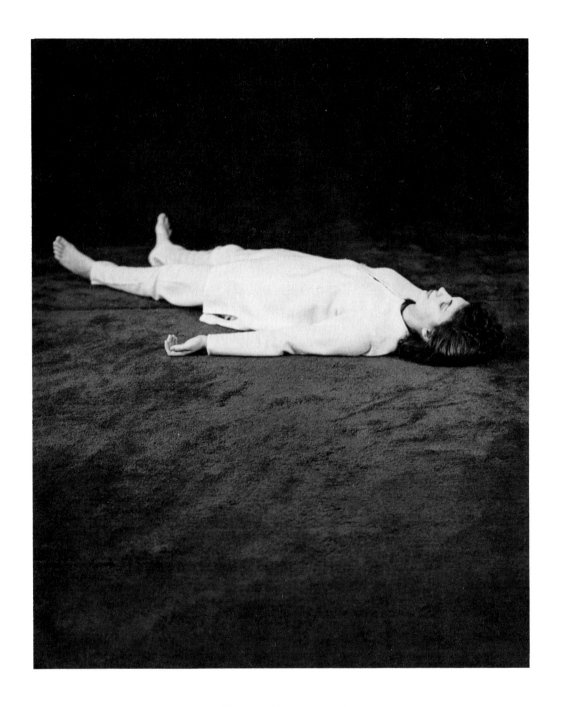

CORPSE (*Shavasana*)

CROCODILE (*Makarasana*)

Lie on your stomach, placing the legs a comfortable distance apart and pointing the toes outward. Fold the arms in front of the body, resting the hands on the upper arms and the forehead on the forearms. Position the elbows and lower arms so that the chest does not touch the floor.

Concentrate on the breath and observe the effects of diaphragmatic breathing. While inhaling, feel the abdominal muscles gently press against the floor; while exhaling, feel the abdominal pressure decrease slightly. Let the body relax completely.

NOTE: If you find it uncomfortable to point the feet outward, you may turn them inward.

Benefits:

- Excellent for relaxation, particularly before and between the prone backward-bending postures.

- This position not only necessitates diaphragmatic breathing, it also teaches you how it feels to breathe diaphragmatically. When you inhale you feel the abdomen press against the floor; when you exhale you feel the abdominal muscles relax. Diaphragmatic breathing causes this same abdominal movement in all positions; however, while you are lying in the crocodile posture, the movement cannot go unnoticed.

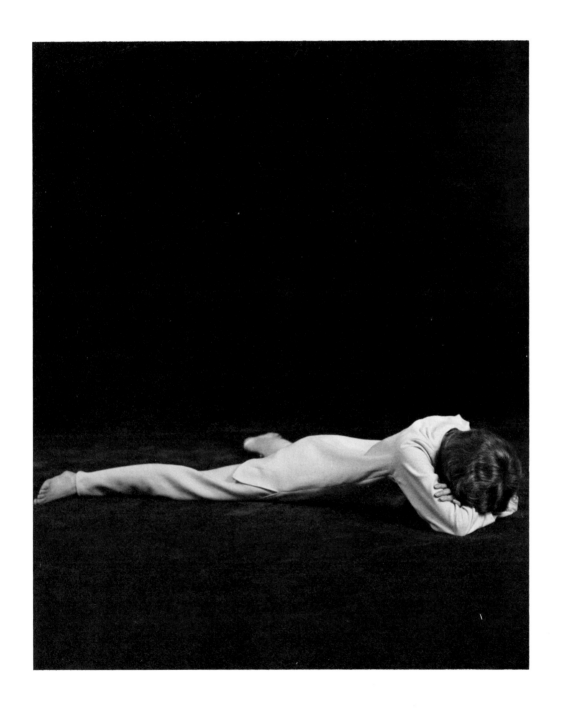

CROCODILE (*Makarasana*)

CHILD'S POSTURE (*Balasana*)

Sit in a kneeling position with the top of the feet on the floor and the buttocks resting on the heels. Keep the head, neck, and trunk straight. Relax the arms and rest the hands on the floor, with the palms upward and fingers pointing behind you.

Exhaling, slowly bend forward from the hips until the stomach and chest rest on the thighs and the forehead touches the floor in front of the knees. As the body bends forward, slide the hands back into a comfortable position.

In the child's posture the body is completely relaxed and very compact. Do not lift the thighs or buttocks off the legs. Keep the arms close to the body. If you experience discomfort, extend the arms above the head a shoulders' width apart. Keep the arms straight and place the palms on the floor. Do not hold this posture for more than five minutes, as it reduces the circulation in the legs. People with excess weight may find this exercise more comfortable if the knees are spread apart.

To release the posture, inhale as you slowly lift the head and trunk and return to a kneeling position.

Benefits:
- Relieves pain in the lower back from minor injury to muscles and ligaments.
- Relaxes the back and promotes healing of more serious injuries, taking pressure off the intervertebral discs by providing a mild and natural form of traction.
- Relieves strain in the lower back, particularly from forward-bending postures.

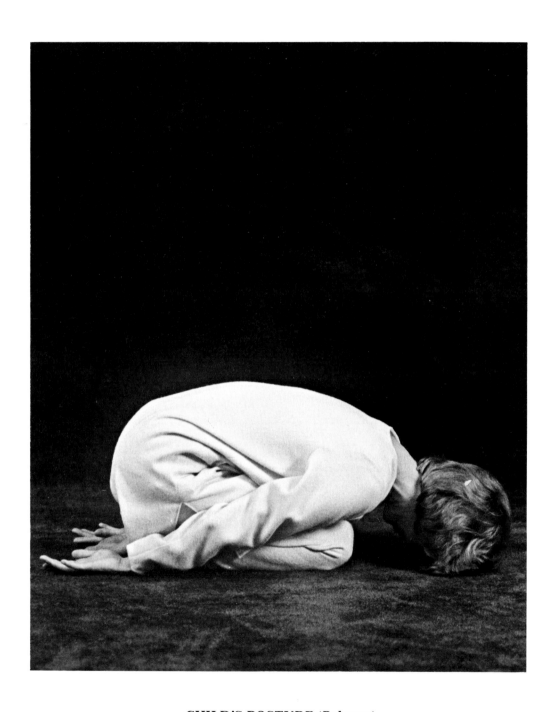

CHILD'S POSTURE (*Balasana*)

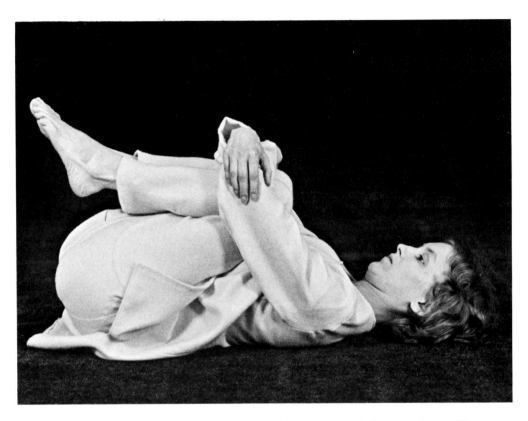

KNEES-TO-CHEST POSTURE

Lie on the back. Bend the legs at the knees and bring them to the chest. Wrap the arms around the legs, pulling them closer toward the chest. The head remains on the floor.

This posture is excellent for relieving strain in the lower back, particularly from the backward-bending and inverted postures. You should hold the posture until this tension is released. Experiment in the posture by gently rocking back and forth or from side to side; hold the posture to one side and then to the other—or simply hold the posture as described above. Discover which position best releases tension at any given time.

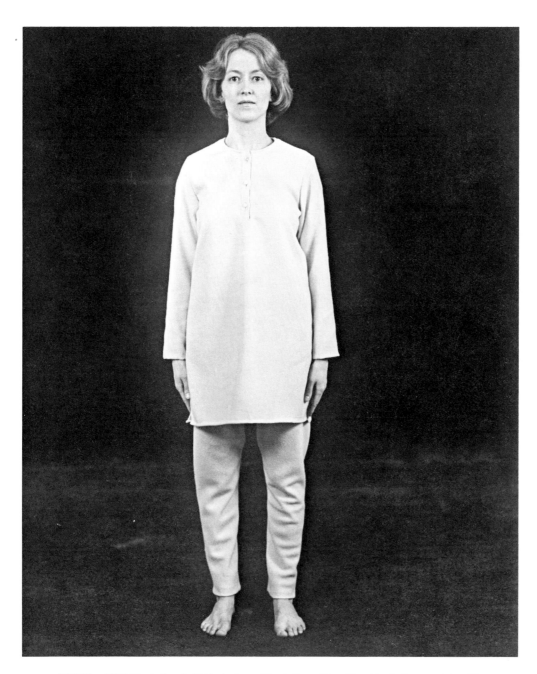

SIMPLE STANDING POSTURE

Stand firmly with the feet 6 to 12 inches apart. Keep the head, neck, and trunk in a straight line and relax the arms and hands at the sides of the body. Breathe evenly.

STRETCHING AND LIMBERING EXERCISES

SYMMETRICAL STRETCH

In this posture the emphasis is on stretching and aligning the vertebrae.

Lie on the floor; place the legs together with the heels and toes touching. With arms overhead and the palms together, inhaling, stretch the torso in an upward direction and the legs in a downward direction, keeping the body symmetrical.

Breathe evenly and hold the body in a stretched position for ten seconds.

Exhaling, simultaneously release the stretch from the toes to the hips and from the fingertips back down to the base of the spine.

Relax and observe the breath.

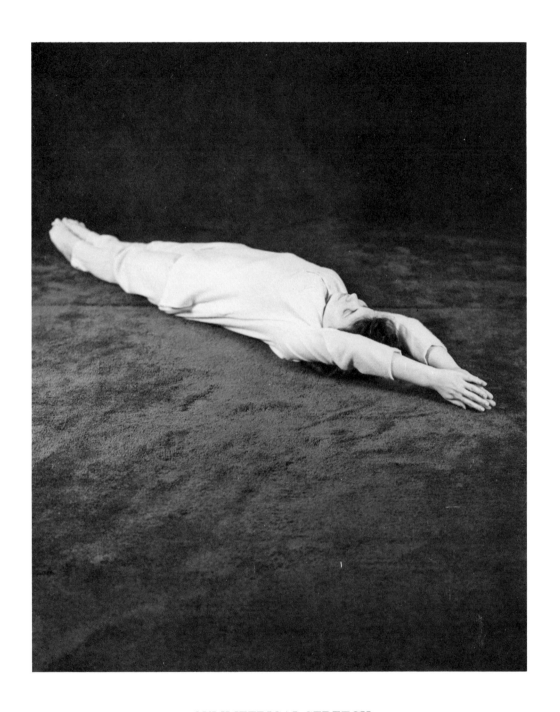

SYMMETRICAL STRETCH

CAT STRETCH

A. Kneel on all fours with the arms straight and a shoulders' width apart; keep the back parallel to the floor, with the knees apart, directly under the hips. The neck should be relaxed with the face toward the floor.

B. Begin exhaling slowly, taking the chin to the chest, allowing the back to arch upward, and pulling the buttocks in.

C. With a slow inhalation, raise the head, stretching through the neck as far as possible. Expand the chest and arch the back downward, stretching the buttocks up.

Then exhaling, slowly lower the head, relax the back, and return to position A.

Relax; then repeat sequence A–B–C–A two more times.

Once the sequence A–B–C–A can be done comfortably, practice the sequence A–B–C–D–E–A, moving smoothly from one position to the next, coordinating each movement with the breath. Note that in the full sequence, you do not return to position A following position C, but instead go directly from position C to position D.

D. Exhaling, slowly lower the head and bend the right knee, bringing it as close as possible to the forehead, while you arch the back upward and stretch it.

E. Inhaling, keeping the hips parallel to the floor, extend the right leg up and back, raise the head as far back as possible, and expand the chest. Feel the stretch through the neck, back, and leg.

Exhaling, slowly lower the leg and head, and return to position A.

Repeat the series, doing positions D and E with the left leg.

NOTE: Each position can also be done as a separate posture that is held while you breathe evenly.

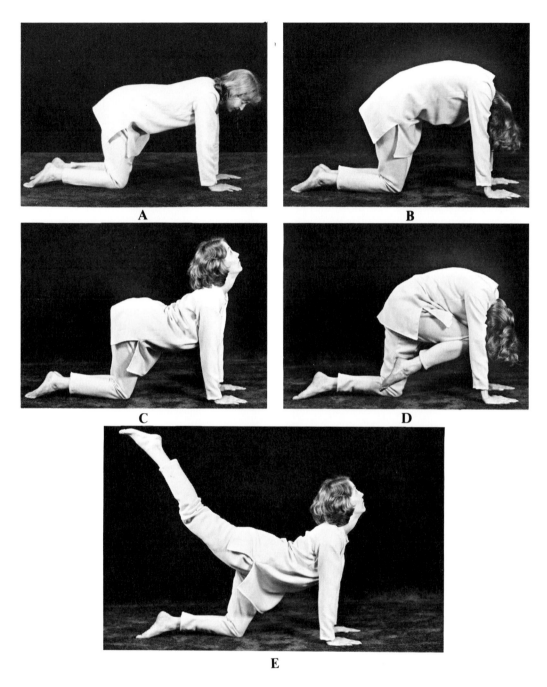

A

B

C

D

E

CAT STRETCH

27

HORIZONTAL STRETCH

Assume the simple standing posture.

Inhale and slowly raise the arms to shoulder level with the palms facing downward. Breathe evenly.

Stretch progressively from the chest, to the shoulders, the upper arms, the elbows, the lower arms, the wrists, the hands, the fingers, and the fingertips. Stretch as far as possible.

Keeping the arms in the same position, slowly relax from the fingertips to the chest.

Exhale and slowly lower the arms and return to the simple standing posture. Concentrate on the breath until the body relaxes completely.

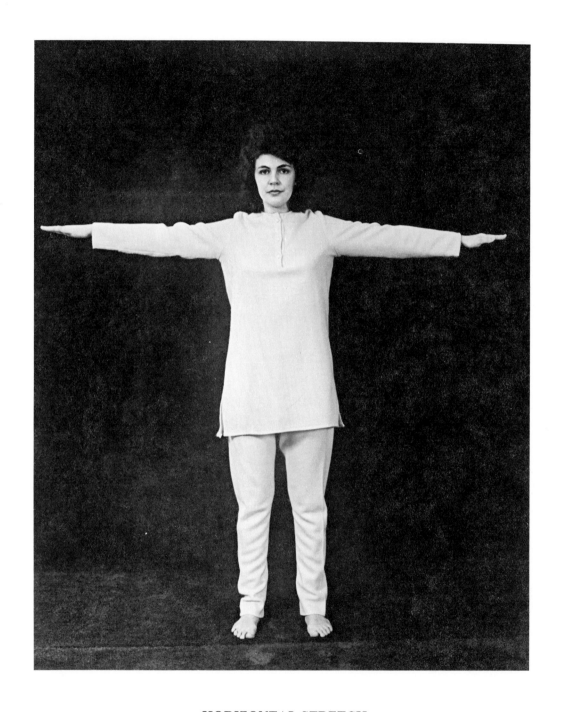

HORIZONTAL STRETCH

OVERHEAD STRETCH

FIRST POSITION

Assume the simple standing posture.

Begin inhaling and slowly raise the arms out to the sides with the palms facing downward. When the arms reach shoulder level, smoothly turn the palms upward. Continue inhaling and raise the arms above the head; place them a shoulders' width apart, with the palms facing each other. (This basic method of raising the arms overhead will be used when practicing the other stretching exercises, unless otherwise stated.)

Keeping the feet firmly on the floor, and breathing evenly, stretch the body upward. Stretch progressively from the lower legs, to the upper legs, the abdomen, the stomach, the chest, the shoulders, the upper arms, the lower arms, the hands, the fingers, and the fingertips.

Keep the arms overhead and slowly relax downward from the fingertips to the feet. Then exhale as you slowly lower the arms. At shoulder level, turn the palms downward and return to the simple standing posture. Concentrate on the breath until the body relaxes completely.

SECOND POSITION

Raise the arms as described above, but this time, after raising the arms, bring the upper arms next to the ears and place the palms together in the prayer position.

Progressively stretch and relax the body as described in the overhead stretch.

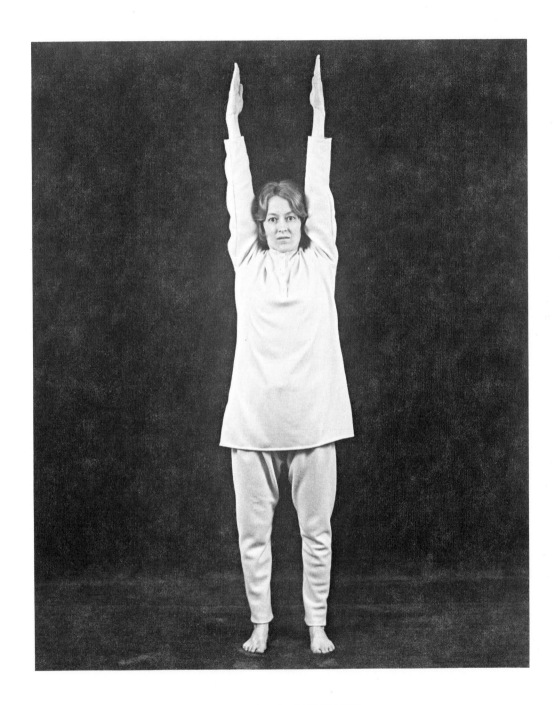

OVERHEAD STRETCH
FIRST POSITION

31

SIDE STRETCH

Assume the simple standing posture with the feet 6 to 12 inches apart.

Begin inhaling and slowly raise the right arm out to the side with the palm facing downward. When the arm reaches shoulder level, turn the palm upward. Continue inhaling and raise the arm until it is next to the ear.

Keeping the feet firmly on the floor, stretch the entire right side of the body upward. Do not allow the body to bend forward or backward or the right arm to bend.

Begin exhaling and slowly bend at the waist, sliding the left hand down the left leg. Breathe evenly for three breaths.

Inhaling, slowly bring the body back to an upright position.

Exhaling, slowly lower the arm to shoulder level, turn the palm downward, and return to the simple standing posture. Concentrate on the breath until the body relaxes completely.

Repeat the side stretch in the opposite direction.

NOTE: For a more intense stretch, repeat this posture with the legs together.

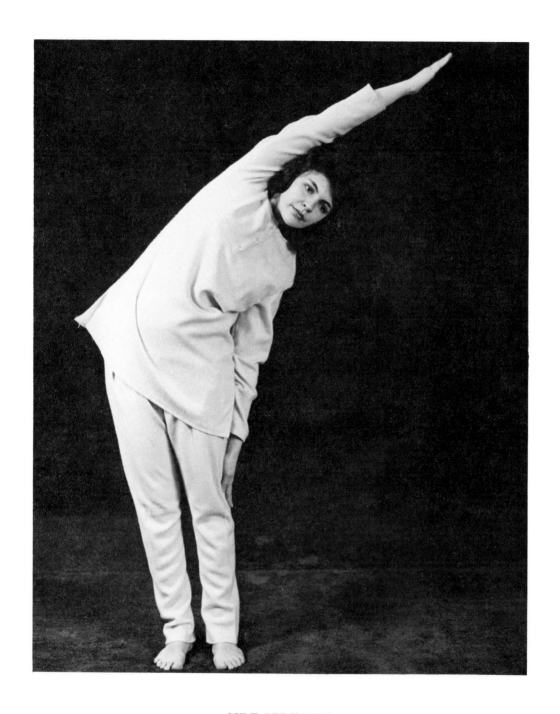

SIDE STRETCH

SIMPLE BACK STRETCH

FIRST POSITION

Assume the simple standing posture.

With the fingers facing downward, place the heels of the hands on either side of the spine just above the buttocks.

Exhaling, stretch up from the base of the spine, and then without pushing the hips forward, slowly bend the head, neck, and trunk backward as far as possible without straining.

Inhaling, return to the standing pose, keeping the hands in the same position.

SECOND POSITION

Place the hands on either side of the spine directly below the rib cage. Repeat the stretch as described in the first position.

RELAXATION POSITION

This forward bend balances the effects of the backward bend.

Begin in the simple standing posture. Keeping the entire body relaxed, slowly bend the body forward as far as possible. Place the hands on the floor or fold the arms and rest each hand in the crook of the opposite arm.

Breathing evenly, hold this position until all the muscles of the back relax completely. Then inhale and return to the standing position.

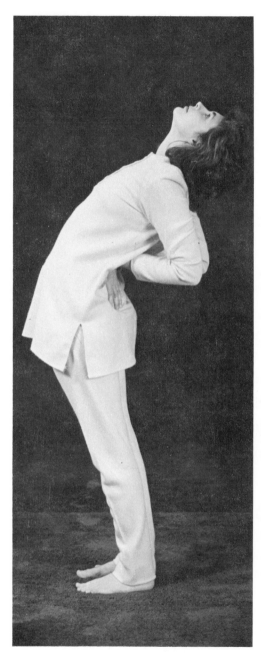 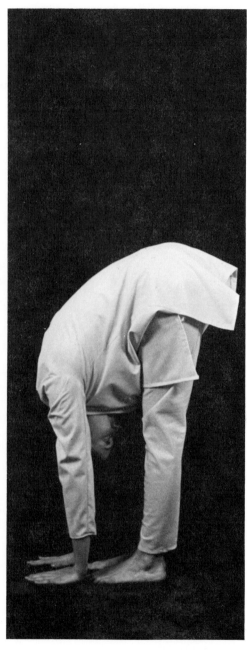

FIRST POSITION   **RELAXATION POSITION**

SIMPLE BACK STRETCH

TORSO TWIST

FIRST POSITION

Assume the simple standing posture with the feet approximately 12 inches apart.

Begin inhaling and slowly raise the arms out to the sides with the palms facing downward. When the arms reach shoulder level, smoothly turn the palms upward. Continue inhaling and raise the arms above the head; place them a shoulders' width apart, with the palms facing each other.

Keeping the arms next to the ears and stretching the body from the rib cage upward, rotate the upper torso and arms in a clockwise direction.

Inhale as the body leans from the front to the right and then to the back; exhale as the body leans to the left and then to the front.

Repeat three times clockwise and then three times counterclockwise.

NOTE: In this position the waist, hips, and legs remain stationary.

SECOND POSITION

Assume the simple standing posture, but with the feet approximately 2 feet apart. Place the hands at the sides of the waist and bend from the waist, repeating the above exercise three times clockwise and three times counterclockwise.

THIRD POSITION

Assume the simple standing posture, but with the feet 2 to 3 feet apart. Keeping the legs stationary, place the hands at the sides of the waist and bending from the hips as far as possible, rotate and twist the entire upper part of the body in a large circle. Repeat three times clockwise and three times counterclockwise. This exercise can also be practiced with the arms overhead, fingers interlaced.

Relax. Concentrate on the breath.

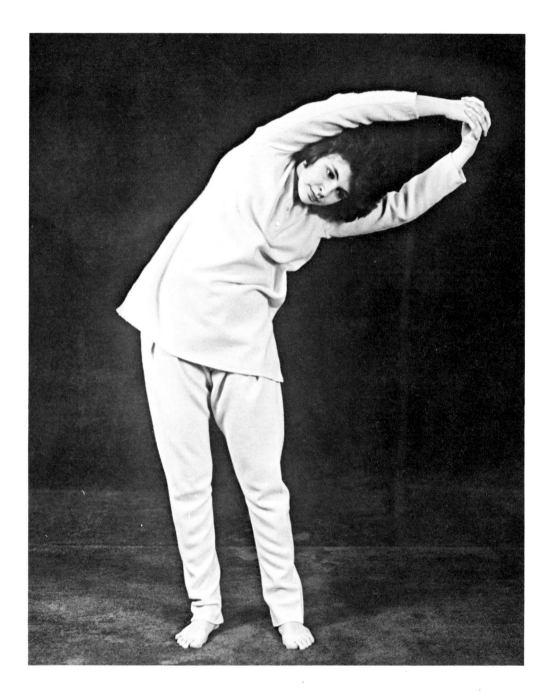

TORSO TWIST
FIRST POSITION

SWIMMING STRETCH

Assume the simple standing posture, but with the feet approximately 3 feet apart.

Inhaling, with one smooth motion raise the arms overhead close to the ears with the palms facing forward.

Exhaling, slowly start lowering the trunk toward the right foot. Breathe evenly while moving the arms and shoulders imitating a swimming motion, alternately stretching first one side of the body and then the other. Bring the head toward the right knee and the hands toward the right foot as far as possible.

Continuing the same swimming motion, slowly return to a standing posture.

Repeat, lowering the trunk toward the left leg. Slowly return to standing.

Repeat, lowering the trunk straight forward. Return to standing.

Relax.

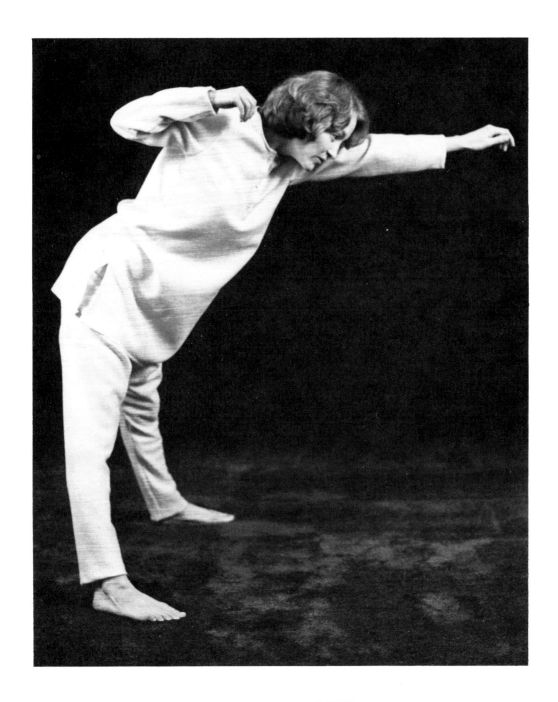

SWIMMING STRETCH

CHURNING (*Chalan*)

Sit on the floor with the head, neck, and trunk straight, with the arms relaxed alongside the body, and the legs extended in front of the body and as far apart as possible. Breathe evenly.

Keeping the back straight, bend forward from the hips and stretch the right hand toward the left foot, moving the left arm behind the back. Bring the head toward the knee and look back toward the left hand.

Repeat the exercise on the opposite side.

Perform the exercise ten times on each side, rhythmically moving from side to side.

NOTE: To increase the stretch of the forward bend, touch the floor on the outside of the foot (as in the accompanying photograph) rather than touching the toes.

Variation 1: Perform the posture as described above, but with the legs 2 to 3 feet apart.

Variation 2: Perform the postures described above, but with the legs together.

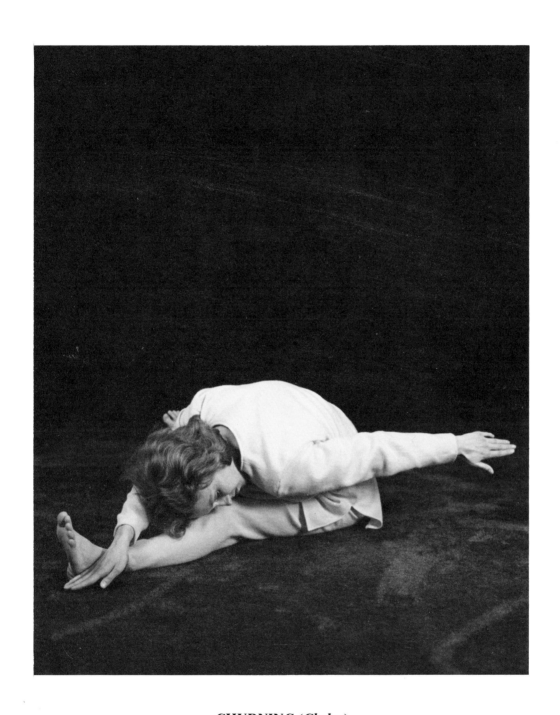

CHURNING (*Chalan*)

41

SUN SALUTATION

SUN SALUTATION
(*Surya Namaskara*)

The sun salutation is a series of twelve positions, each flowing into the next in one graceful, continuous movement. These exercises are performed a few times before beginning the asanas. While facing the rising sun with an attitude of worship, the traditional practitioner silently repeats each movement's seed mantra as he performs it. The sun shines for all and excludes none from its light and life-giving energy. In performing salutations to the sun, we ask for that light and energy to unfold within us.

Although not considered part of traditional yoga postures by many schools of hatha yoga, *surya namaskara* is an excellent warm-up exercise; it stretches and limbers the spine and limbs. While performing surya namaskara, coordinate the twelve positions with the breath; inhale as you go into one position and exhale as you go into the next. Retain the breath only in the fifth position.

At first, practice the entire exercise three times. Practice it slowly without going beyond your capacity. During the first week, become familiar with the movements only. It is important that from position 3 through position 10 the hands remain in the same place. Once you are familiar with the positions, you can coordinate the breathing and body movements. The sun salutation sets the proper mood of inner and outer harmony essential to the true practice and goal of hatha yoga.

After performing surya namaskara, relax the body completely before beginning your yoga asanas.

The benefits of surya namaskara are numerous. While asleep, the body lies in an inactive condition. During this time, the conscious mind ceases to function, the metabolic rate decreases, the circulation of the body fluids slows, and the functional capacity of the rest of the body lessens considerably. Upon awakening, the body and mind must make a transition from this inactive condition to one of activity. Surya namaskara aids in this transition by massaging and stimulating the glands, organs, muscles, and nerves of the body. The breath rate increases, bringing more oxygen into the lungs, thus quickening the heart rate. This in turn causes more blood to pass through the lungs, picking up oxygen, and therefore, sending a greater supply of oxygenated blood throughout the different parts of the body.

The movements in the sun salutation incorporate four asanas: the back-bending posture (*urdhvasana*), positions 2 and 11; the hand-to-foot posture (*padahastasana*), positions 3 and 10; the cobra posture (*bhujangasana*), position 7; and the dog-stretch posture (*adho mukha shvanasana*), position 8. Of course, the benefits of each of these postures are not as great when the postures are performed as part of the sun salutation as they are when the postures are performed separately and held for a longer time.

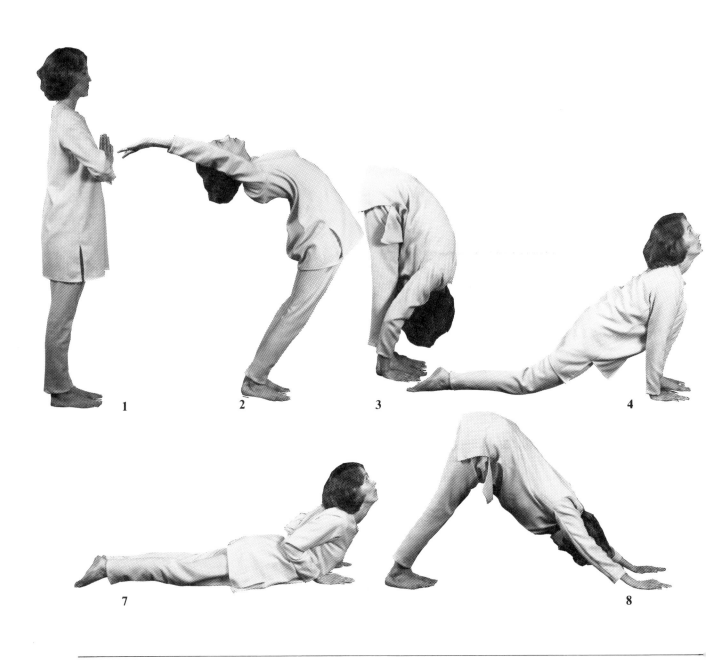

WITH HANDS IN PRAYER I FACE THE SUN, FEELING LOVE AND JOY IN MY

BEFORE THE SUN'S RADIANCE AND PLACE MY FACE TO THE GROUND IN

TO ACHIEVE SUCH HEIGHTS, I MUST BE AS THE DUST OF THE EARTH.   I

AND AGAIN SURRENDER.   I STAND TALL AS I REMEMBER THE TRUE SUN

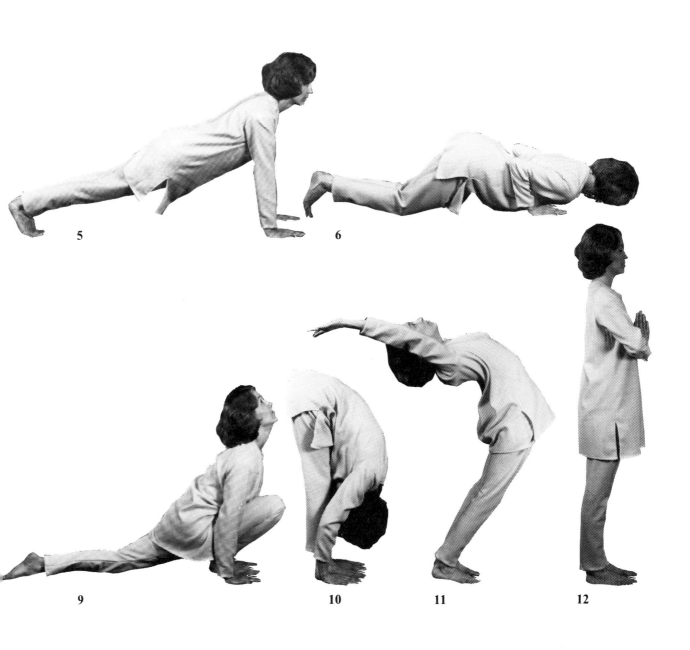

HEART.   I REACH OUT AND LET THE SUN FILL ME WITH WARMTH. I BOW

HUMBLE RESPECT.   I LIFT MY FACE TO THE SUN AND THEN REMEMBER,

STRETCH UP TOWARDS ITS LIGHT TRYING TO REACH THE GREATEST HEIGHTS

IS WITHIN ME.

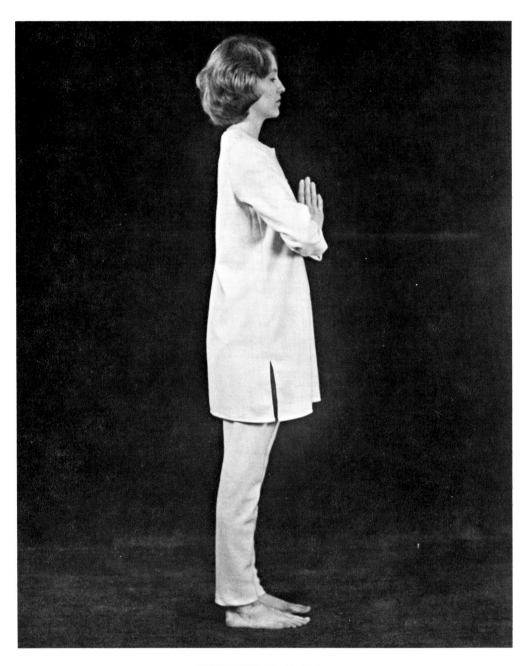

POSITION 1: Exhale

Stand firmly with the head, neck, and trunk in a straight line. Beginners can stand with the feet slightly apart. With palms together in prayer position, place the hands before the heart and gently close the eyes. Standing silently, concentrate on the breath and mentally repeat a short positive affirmation.

48

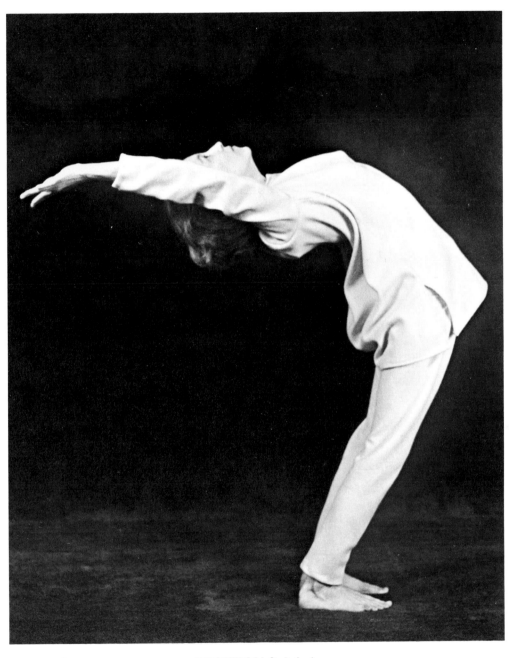

POSITION 2: Inhale

Inhaling, slightly lower and stretch the hands and arms forward with the palms facing downward. Raise the arms overhead until they are next to the ears. Keeping the legs straight, and the head between the arms, arch the spine and bend backward as far as possible without straining. (An alternative method for beginning students is to bend backward only as far as possible without thrusting the hips forward.)

49

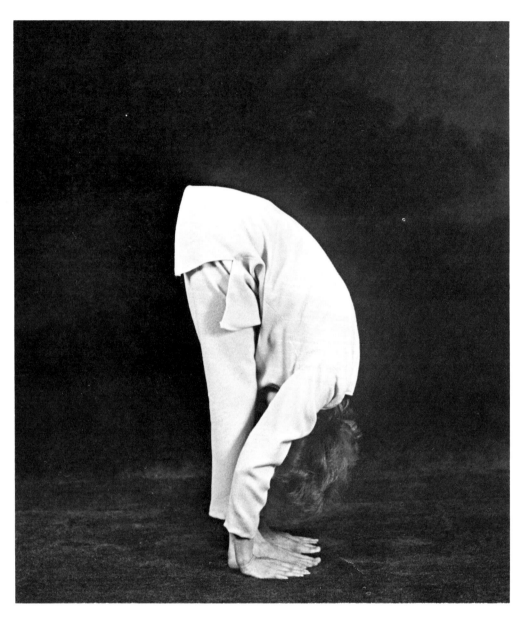

POSITION 3: Exhale

Exhaling, bend forward from the hips, keeping the back straight and the arms next to the ears. Continue bending; place the palms next to the feet, aligning the fingers with the toes. Bring the head to the knees, keeping the legs straight.

NOTE: If you cannot place the hands on the floor without bending the legs, lower the hands only as far as possible without straining. Then to go into position 4, first bend the knees and place the hands on the floor next to the feet.

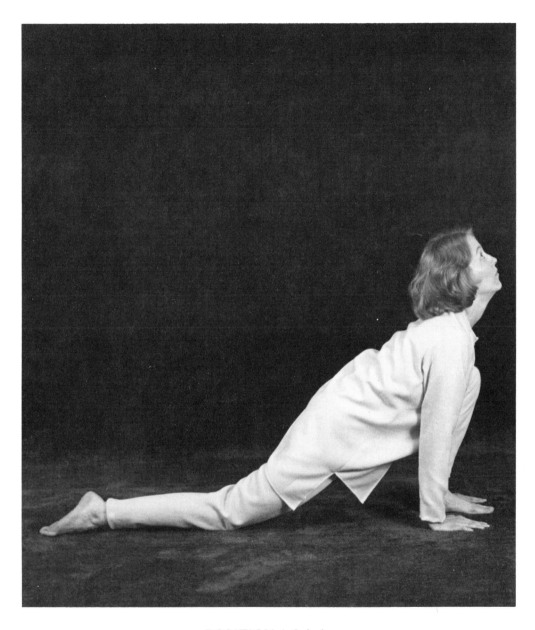

POSITION 4: Inhale

Inhaling, stretch the right leg back, rest the right knee and the top of the right foot on the floor, and extend the toes. The left foot remains between the hands; the hands remain firmly on the floor. Arch the back, look up, and stretch the head back as far as possible. The line from the head to the tip of the right foot should form a smooth and graceful curve.

NOTE: When performing multiple sun salutations, the fore and aft legs should be alternated.

51

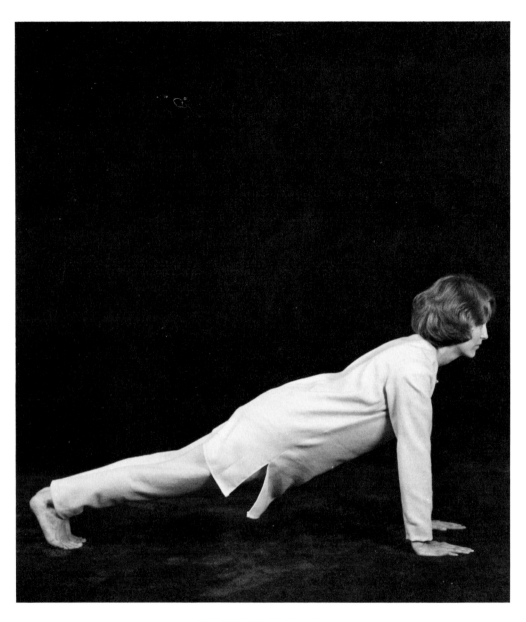

POSITION 5: Retain

Retain the breath. (This is the only position in which the breath is held.) Curl the toes of the right foot; extend the left leg, placing it next to the right. The arms remain straight and the body forms an inclined plane from the head to the feet. This position resembles a starting push-up position.

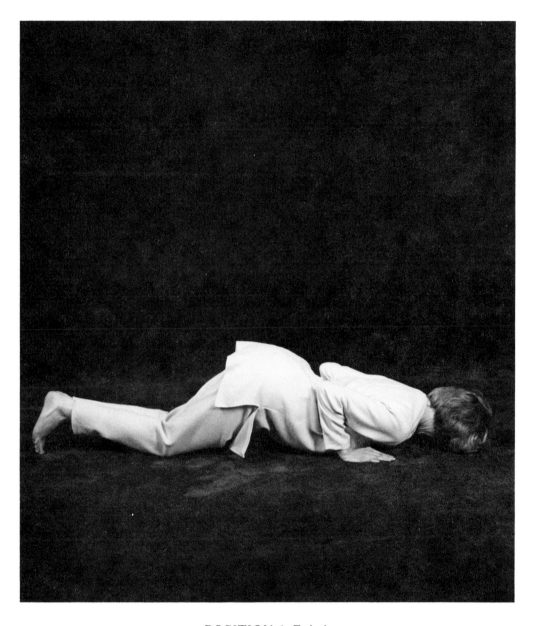

POSITION 6: Exhale

Exhaling, drop first the knees and then the chest to the floor, keeping the tips of the fingers in line with the breasts. Tuck in the chin and place the forehead on the floor.

In this position only the toes, knees, hands, chest, and forehead touch the floor. Neither the nose nor the chin should touch the floor. The elbows should remain close to the body.

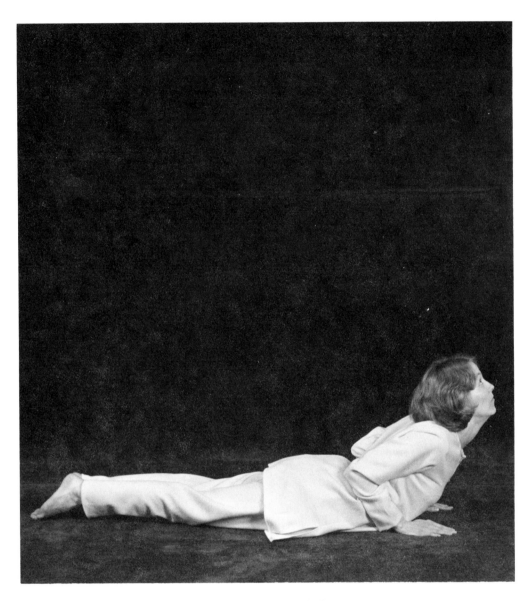

POSITION 7: Inhale

Without moving the hands and forehead, relax the legs and extend the feet so that the body rests flat on the floor. Inhaling, slowly begin to raise the head. First, touch the nose and then the chin to the floor; then, stretch the head forward and upward. Without using the strength of the arms or hands, slowly raise the shoulders and chest; look up and bend back as far as possible.

In this posture the navel remains on the floor. To lift the thorax, use the muscles of the back only. Do not use the arms and hands to push the body off the floor, but only to balance the body. Keep the feet and legs together and relaxed.

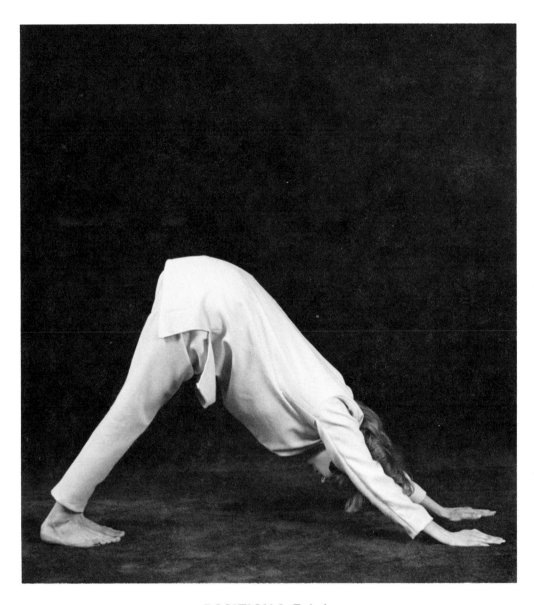

POSITION 8: Exhale

Without repositioning the feet and hands, exhaling, press the feet to the floor so that the toes point toward the hands; straighten the arms, pushing the buttocks high in the air. Bring the head between the arms and try to press the heels to the floor.

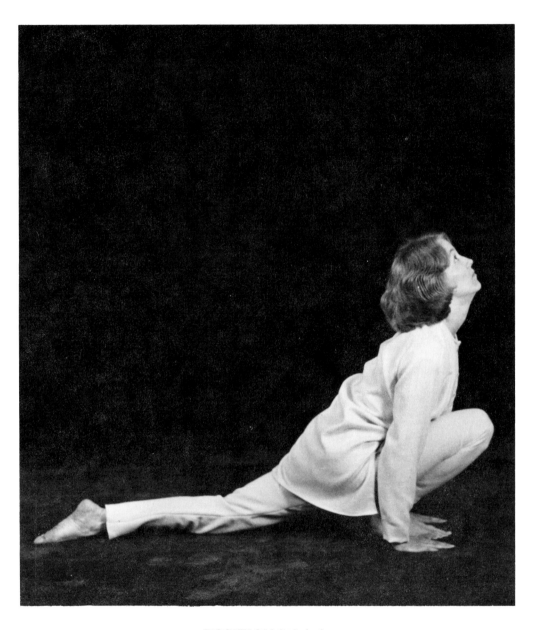

POSITION 9: Inhale

Inhaling, bend the right knee and place the right foot between the hands. Align the toes with the fingers. Rest the left knee and the top of the left foot on the floor and extend the toes. Arch the back, stretch the head back, look up, and bend back as far as possible.

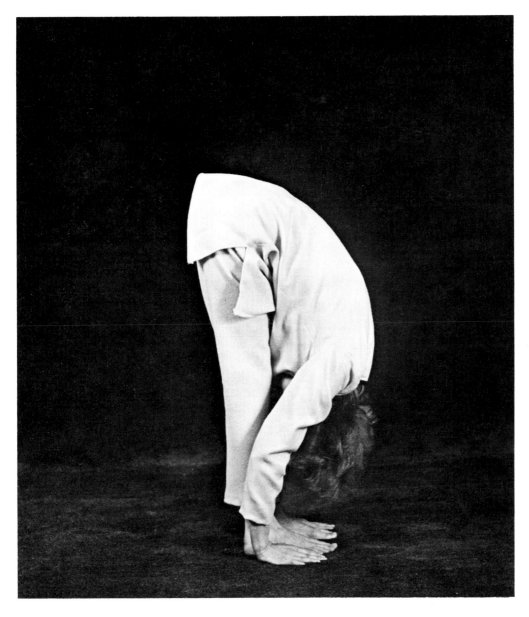

POSITION 10: Exhale

Exhaling, place the left foot beside the right, keeping the palms on the floor. Straighten the legs and bring the head to the knees.

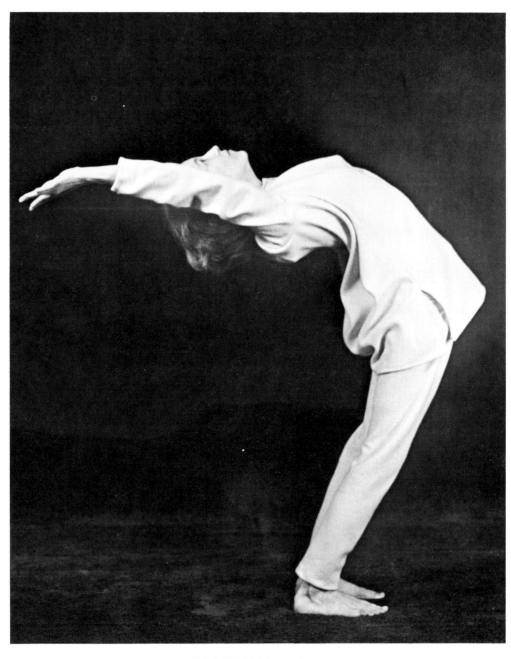

POSITION 11: Inhale

Inhaling, slowly raise the body, stretching the arms out, up, and back; bend back as far as possible without straining. Remember to keep the arms close to the ears and the legs straight.

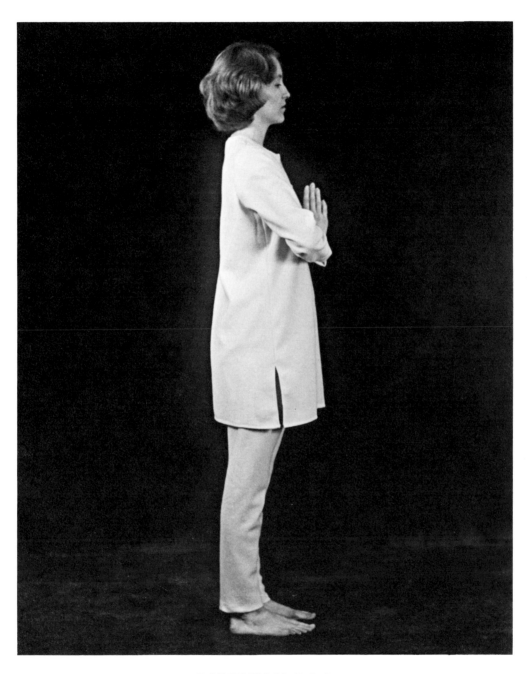

POSITION 12: Exhale

Exhaling, return to an erect standing position. Slowly lower the arms and bring the hands to the chest in prayer position.

ASANAS AND PREPARATORY EXERCISES

Asanas

"Asanas make one firm, free from maladies, and light of limb."

—*Hathayogapradipika* of Svatmarama, Chapter 1, Verse 17

The benefits and purposes of the asanas may be concisely summarized as follows. First, to prepare the body for meditation, making it calm, steady, and firm. Second, to free the body from disease (dis-ease); to develop superb health so that the mind is not distracted by aches and pains after the body has been made steady for meditation. Third, to bring lightness to the body—not only literally, by reducing excess weight and increasing suppleness, but also figuratively, counteracting heaviness and depression by developing lightness of feeling and expression.

The postures benefit primarily the vertebral column and internal organs. Almost every posture either involves back-bending in one direction or another or entails carefully focusing the mind on maintaining a perfect posture. In addition to the direct effects of developing a healthy spine, the bending and twisting postures also have important effects on the internal organs. These postures supplement the constant movement and gentle massaging of the viscera (the internal organs) that occur with diaphragmatic breathing. For example, many of the bending and twisting postures cause an increase in intra-abdominal pressure, which in turn forces stagnant venous blood out of the internal organs, thereby encouraging the perfusion of the organs with arterial blood.

The inverted postures have important effects on both circulation and respiration. A large pool of venous blood in the legs normally depends on muscular activity to pump the blood past valves and back to the heart—activity that is sadly deficient in many people in our society. The upside-down postures quickly drain this blood from the legs and improve circulation. The diaphragm is our most important muscle of respiration, but is frequently misused and almost universally underused. You can quickly learn diaphragmatic breathing in a mild upside-down posture, such as the inverted action posture, because the weight of the abdominal organs pushes the diaphragm to an especially high position in the chest during exhalation. You can relate to this visually by observing the resulting cavitation on the front side of the abdomen. During inhalation, the diaphragm must then push the abdominal organs up, against the force of gravity, and this in turn pushes out the abdominal wall, again providing visual feedback that is easily observable.

All the postures help in preparing for meditation. Most of us when we first begin to practice meditation find that sitting in a comfortable and easy posture with the head, neck, and trunk straight is an impossibility. Many years of bad habits, influences, and attitudes have encourged us to develop poor posture. This can result in physical ailments such as low back pain, excessive fatigue, and incorrect and shallow breathing. Systematically practicing the various postures and breathing exercises in this manual will greatly aid you in strengthening the muscles of the back, in stretching and limbering the other muscles and ligaments of the body, and in improving flexibility of the joints, thereby preparing you for the practice of meditation.

Benefits are also listed for many of the individual postures. These comments are the culmination of thousands of years of self-observation by teachers and students who have devoted their lives to understanding the working of the human body. Full appreciation and understanding of the effects of the posture can never be achieved unless the postures are practiced. Your own body is the finest laboratory imaginable, and nothing can substitute for the direct personal knowledge that is the primary tradition of this science.

A. STANDING POSTURES

ABDOMINAL LIFT
(*Uddiyana Bandha*)

Stand with the feet approximately 2 feet apart. Keeping the spine straight, bend the knees slightly, and lean forward from the waist only far enough to place the palms of the hands just above the knees. Be sure the head remains above the hips.

Exhale completely and place the chin on the hollow of the throat. (The chin lock is not shown in the accompanying photograph.)

Without inhaling, suck the abdominal muscles in and up, pulling the navel toward the spine. This motion pulls the diaphragm up and creates a cavity on the front side of the abdomen under the rib cage.

Hold this position without inhaling as long as it remains comfortable. Then slowly release the abdominal muscles while inhaling, return to an erect standing position, and relax.

Use force only in pulling the abdominal muscles in; **never** force the muscles outward.

Do not practice this exercise if you have high blood pressure, a hiatal hernia, ulcers, or a heart disorder. Women should not practice it during menstruation or pregnancy, or if using an IUD.

Benefits:

- Promotes health in all the internal organs.

- Stimulates digestion.

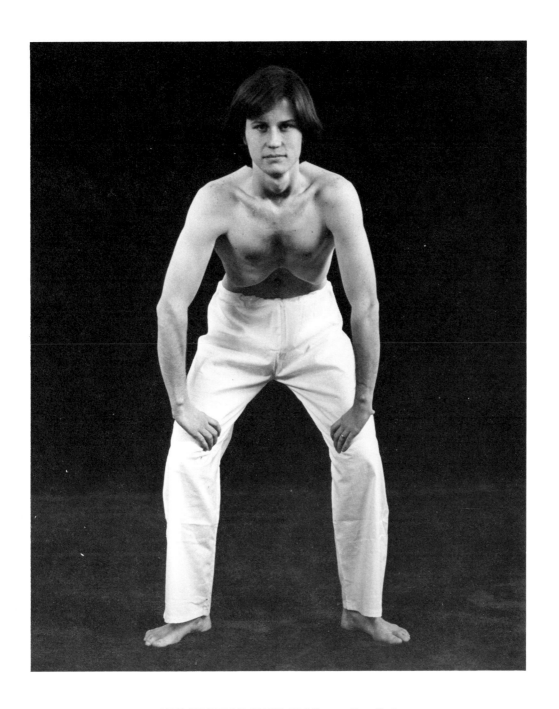

ABDOMINAL LIFT (*Uddiyana Bandha*)

ANGLE POSTURE (*Konasana*)

FIRST POSITION

Assume the simple standing posture, but with the feet 2 to 3 feet apart.

Placing the arms behind the back, grasp the right wrist with the left hand. Keep the heels in line and place the right foot at a 90° angle from the left. (Beginning students may turn the left foot slightly inward [to the right] if that is more comfortable.) Turn the body toward the right foot.

Exhaling, bend forward from the hips, keeping the head up and the back straight. Come as far down as you can with the back straight, then allow the head to drop as close to the knee as possible, relaxing the back. Breathe evenly for 3 breaths.

Inhaling, slowly raise the body to an upright position and arch the back slightly. Exhaling, turn to the front. Turn the right foot so that it faces forward.

Repeat on the left side.

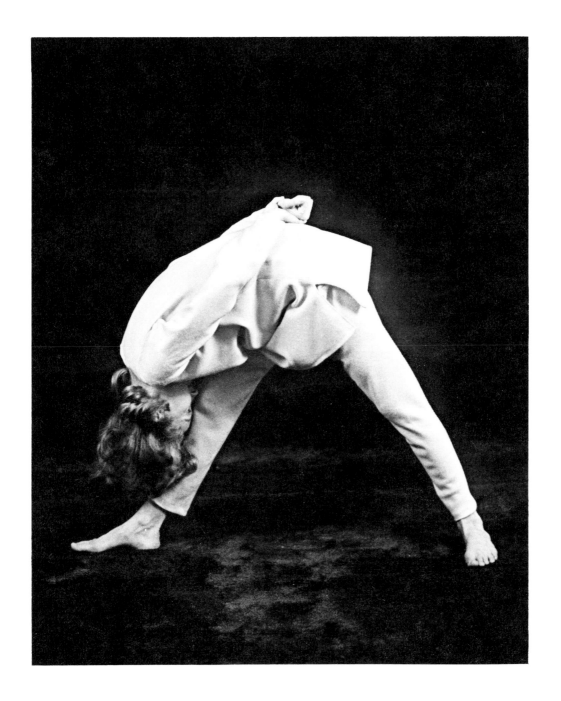

ANGLE POSTURE (*Konasana*)
FIRST POSITION

SECOND POSITION

Assume the simple standing posture, but with the feet 2 to 3 feet apart. Interlace the fingers behind the back.

Inhaling, lift the chin and arch back slightly.

Exhaling, bend forward from the hips, keeping the head up and the back straight. Come as far down as you can with the back straight, then allow the head to come down between the legs. Raise the arms overhead. Breathe evenly; hold for three breaths.

Inhaling, slowly raise the body, simultaneously allowing the hands to lower behind the back, and arch back slightly.

Exhaling, return to an upright position, release the hands and relax.

Arm Variation in Second Position: Repeat the exercise with the fingers interlaced behind the back and the palms pressed together. When arching back before and after the forward bend, push the hands down toward the floor as far as possible.

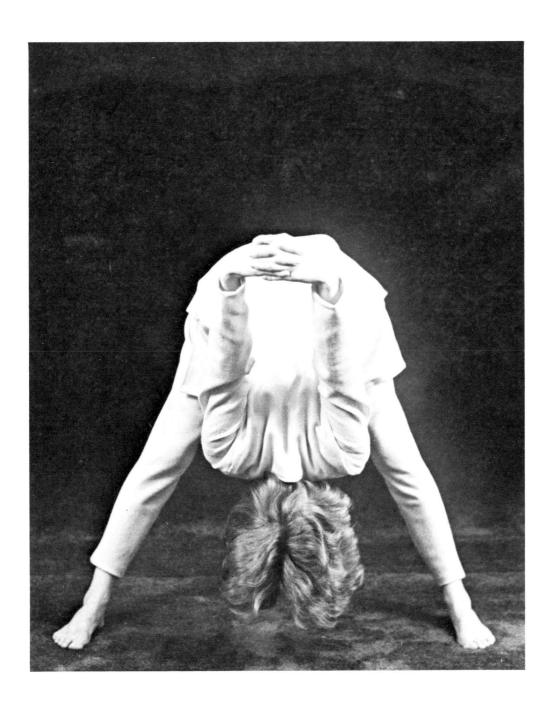

ANGLE POSTURE (*Konasana*)
SECOND POSITION

TRIANGLE (*Trikonasana*)

Assume the simple standing posture, but with the feet 3 feet apart. Keep the heels in line and place the right foot at a 90° angle from the left. (Beginning students may turn the left foot slightly inward [to the right] if that is more comfortable.) Inhaling, slowly raise the arms away from your sides to shoulder level with the palms facing downward.

Exhaling, and making sure that the hips remain facing forward, lower the torso to the right. Place the right hand on the lower leg, keeping the arms and the legs straight. The arms remain in line with each other, and the left arm extends straight up with the palm facing to the front. The head should be turned to look up at the left hand. Breathe evenly and hold to your comfortable capacity.

Inhaling, slowly return to a standing position and turn the right foot so that it faces forward.

Repeat, bringing the left hand to the left leg.

Inhaling, slowly return to a standing position and turn the left foot so that it faces forward. Exhaling, slowly lower the arms.

Variation 1: Perform the posture as described above, but place the hand on the floor on the inside of the foot.

Variation 2: Perform the posture as described above, but place the hand on the floor on the outside of the foot.

Benefits:

- Increases flexibility of the spinal column and hip joints.

- Lengthens the hamstring muscles on the back of the thighs.

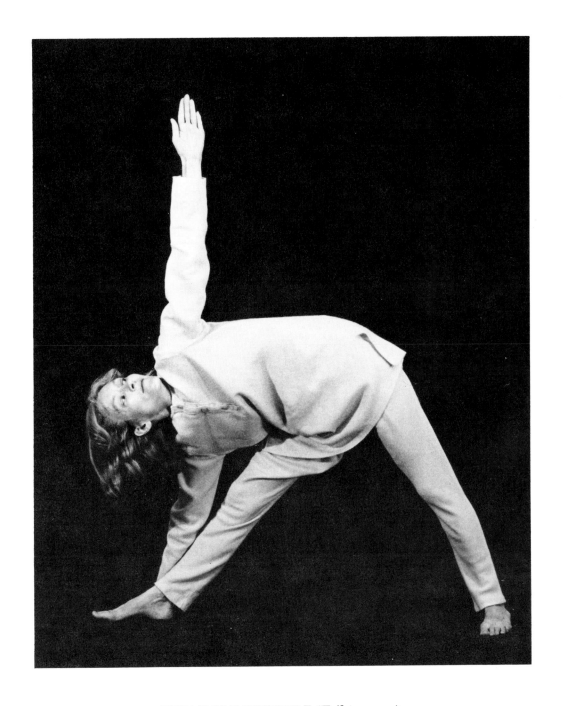

TRIANGLE POSTURE (*Trikonasana*)

PREPARATION FOR REVOLVING TRIANGLE

Assume the simple standing posture, but with the feet 3 feet apart. Keep the heels in line and place the right foot at a 90° angle from the front and the left foot at a 45° angle toward the right. Inhaling, slowly raise the arms away from your sides to shoulder level with the palms facing downward, and stretch from the chest out to the fingertips.

Maintain the stretch through the arms, keeping the arms straight out at shoulder level, and, exhaling, twist the upper torso to the right as far as you can. Turn the head to look over the right shoulder. Breathe evenly and hold to your comfortable capacity. Inhaling, twist back to the front and then turn the feet to face forward.

Repeat, reversing the position of the feet and twisting the torso to the left. Breathe evenly and hold to your comfortable capacity. Inhaling, twist back to the front, and then bring the feet to face forward. Exhaling, slowly lower the arms. Relax.

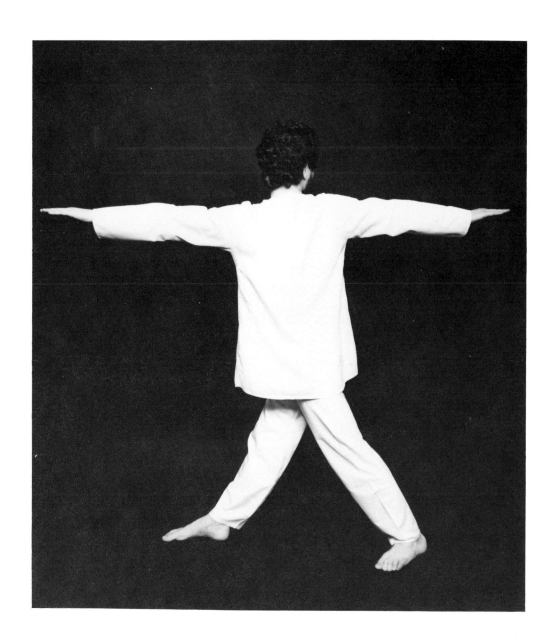

PREPARATION FOR REVOLVING TRIANGLE

REVOLVING TRIANGLE
(*Parivritta Trikonasana*)

Assume the simple standing posture, but with the feet 3 feet apart.

Inhaling, slowly raise the arms away from your sides to shoulder level with the palms facing downward.

Exhaling, gently stretch from the chest out to the fingertips.

Inhaling, twist the upper torso to the right.

Exhaling, bring the left hand to the floor on the inside of the right foot; keep the arms and legs straight. The arms remain in line with each other, and the right arm extends straight up. When the body is steady and comfortable, turn the head and look up at the right hand.

Breathe evenly; hold to your comfortable capacity.

Inhaling, and maintaining the twist in the torso, slowly return to a standing position.

Exhaling, turn back to center.

Repeat, bringing the right hand to the inside of the left foot.

NOTE: If you find it difficult in the beginning to place your hand on the floor, bend forward only as far as you can comfortably and place the hand on the leg or foot. The arms and legs should remain straight at all times.

Variation: Perform the posture as described above, but turning the right foot out at a 90° angle. Beginning students may also turn the left foot slightly inward (to the right) if that is more comfortable. Place the left hand on the floor at the inside of the right foot. The palm of the right hand faces back.

Repeat, bringing the right hand to the inside of the left foot.

Benefits:

- Increases flexibility of the spinal column and hip joints.
- Lengthens the hamstring muscles on the back of the thighs.

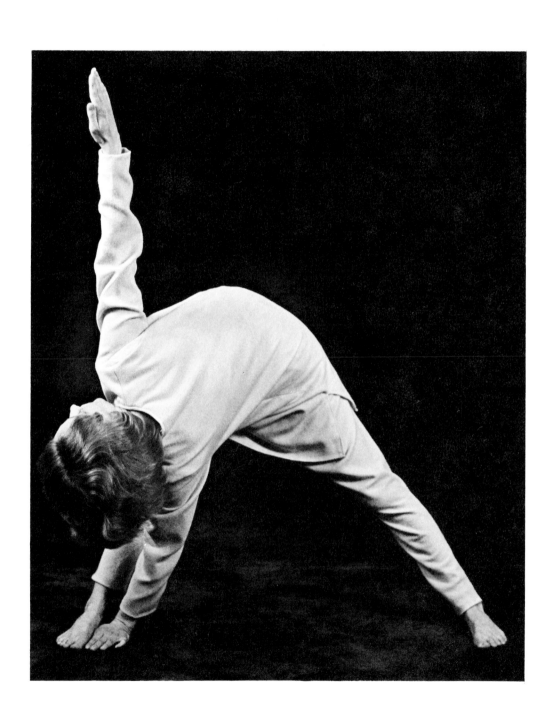

REVOLVING TRIANGLE (*Parivritta Trikonasana*)

TREE (*Vrikshasana*)

FIRST POSITION

Stand erect with the legs together.

Bend the right leg at the knee and slide the right foot up the left leg. Without bending forward, grasp the right ankle with the right hand and position the heel snugly against the perineum (the area between the genitals and the anus). Rest the sole of the foot on the inside of the left thigh, with the knee turned out to the side at a 90° angle.

Balance steadily on the left foot. While inhaling, bring the hands to the chest in a prayer position. Breathe evenly and hold for 15 to 20 seconds. Then lower the hands and arms, and release the foot. Relax, standing on both feet.

Repeat, standing on the right leg.

NOTE: In this posture the body remains balanced and still. You will find it helpful to fix your gaze on a stationary point a few feet away. If you find it too difficult to bring the foot to the thigh, first practice the posture with the foot at the ankle and then the knee.

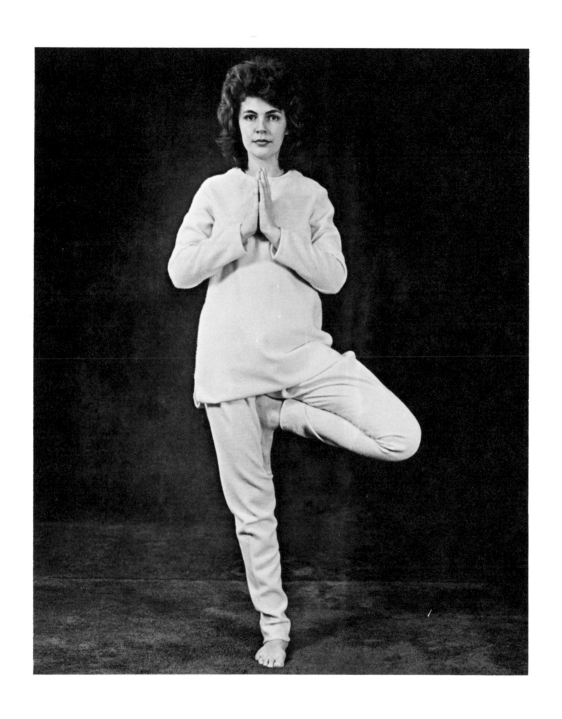

TREE (*Vrikshasana*)

SECOND POSITION

When you feel steady and confident in the first position, raise both arms overhead. Place the palms together, keep the upper arms next to the ears, and stretch the arms upward. Hold for 15 to 20 seconds.

THIRD POSITION

Instead of placing the foot as high on the leg as possible, place it on top of the thigh in the half lotus position. Bring the hands to the chest in a prayer position. Hold for 15 to 20 seconds.

FOURTH POSITION

With the foot on top of the thigh in the half lotus position, stretch the arms overhead and place the palms together. Hold for 15 to 20 seconds.

Benefits:

- Develops poise and concentration, which are helpful for the performance of all postures.

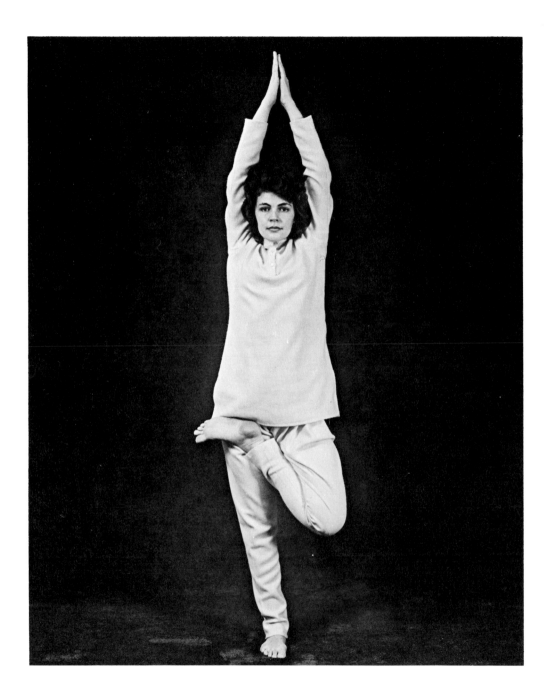

TREE (*Vrikshasana*)
FOURTH POSITION

PREPARATION FOR HAND-TO-FOOT POSTURE

Stand with the head, neck, and trunk straight, feet together. Inhaling, with the palms facing downward, raise the arms in front of the body until they are overhead close to the ears.

Exhaling, bend forward from the hips, keeping the back straight and the arms close to the ears. Come down as far as you can with the back straight, then lower the head, relaxing the neck and shoulders. Take the head as close to the knees as you comfortably can. Fold the arms, grasping the elbows with the hands; keep the legs straight. Breathe evenly; hold for 5 to 10 seconds.

Inhaling, raise the torso, stretching the arms overhead. Exhaling, lower the arms and relax.

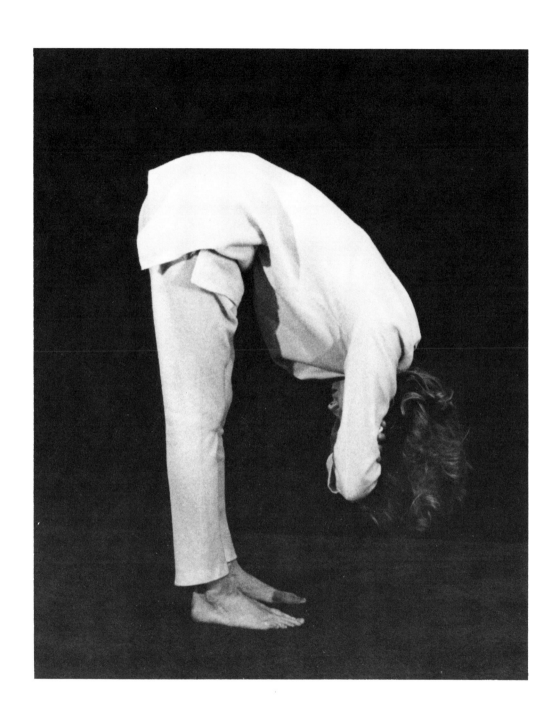

PREPARATION FOR HAND-TO-FOOT POSTURE

HAND-TO-FOOT POSTURE
(*Padahastasana*)

Stand with the head, neck, and trunk in a straight line, feet together.

Inhaling, raise the arms in front of the body until they are overhead close to the ears, with the palms facing forward.

Exhaling, bend forward from the hips, keeping the back straight and the arms close to the ears. Place the palms of the hands on the floor at the sides of the feet. Bring the head to the knees, keeping the legs straight. Breathe evenly; hold for 5 to 10 seconds.

Inhaling, raise the torso, stretching the arms overhead.

Exhaling, lower the arms and relax.

Variation 1: Grasp the back of the ankles with the hands.

Variation 2: Grasp the big toes with the fingers.

Benefits:

- Relieves constipation.

- Decreases excess abdominal fat.

- Makes the spine supple and stretches the hamstring muscles.

NOTE: This posture gives the same benefits as the sitting forward bend; however, beginners often find this posture more useful than the sitting forward bend because in the hand-to-foot posture gravity aids one in moving to one's limit in the posture.

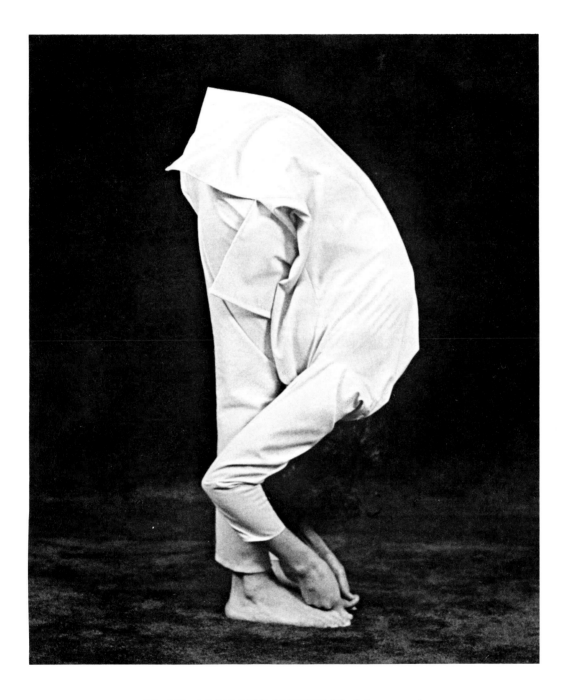

HAND-TO-FOOT POSTURE (*Padahastasana*)
VARIATION 2

B. SITTING POSTURES

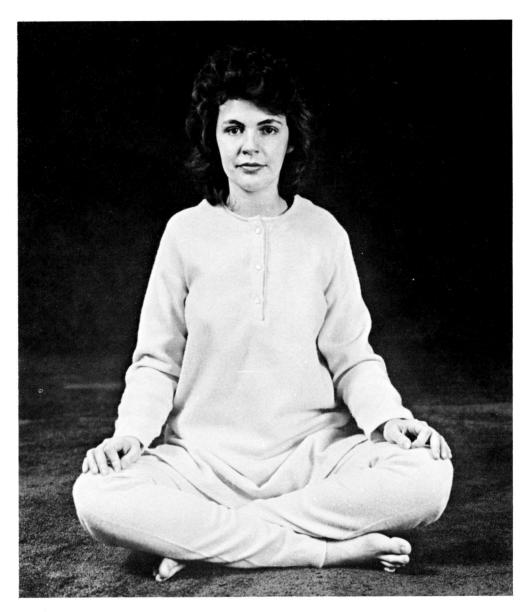

EASY POSTURE (*Sukhasana*)

This is a simple cross-legged posture.

Sit with the head, neck, and trunk straight. Place the left foot beneath the right knee and the right foot beneath the left knee. Each knee rests on the opposite foot.

This posture is useful for beginners and older people, especially if the other sitting postures are painful or uncomfortable.

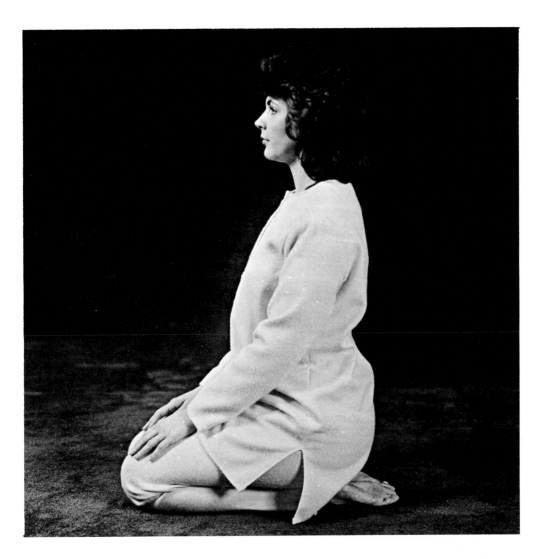

KNEELING POSTURE (*Vajrasana*)

Sit in a kneeling position with the knees together and the head, neck, and trunk straight. Place the hands, palms downward, above the knees.

This sitting posture (also called the Zen posture) is used in two asanas described in this manual: the lion, and a variation of the yoga mudra. It is also useful in developing an awareness of good posture.

CAUTION: It is not recommended that this posture be held for an extended period of time. Injury to the peroneal nerve of the lower leg, which can cause permanent dropping of the foot, may result from staying in the posture too long. Also, persons suffering from varicose veins should avoid this posture.

HALF LOTUS (*Ardha Padmasana*)

This posture is a preparation for the full lotus posture.

Sit with the head, neck, and trunk straight, with the legs together and fully extended in front of you. Bend the right leg, take hold of the foot, and turn it upward. Place the heel firmly against the abdominal wall on the inside of the left hip bone. Bend the left leg and tuck it under the right. Gently bring the right knee toward the floor. Rest the hands on the knees.

Repeat, placing the left leg in the half lotus.

NOTE: Exercise caution in this posture if you have any knee problems.

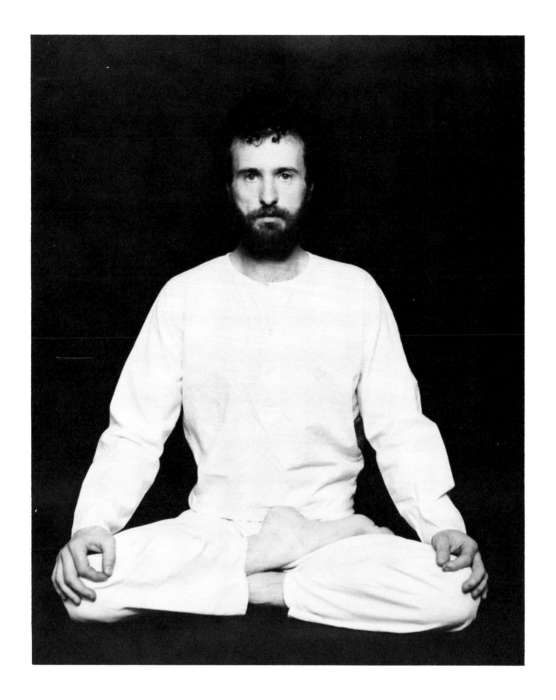

HALF LOTUS (*Ardha Padmasana*)

LEG CRADLES

FIRST POSITION

Sit cross-legged with the head, neck, and trunk straight.

Cradle the left leg, holding the knee with the left hand and holding the foot with the right hand. Gently rock the leg from side to side, moving it from the hip.

Repeat with the right leg.

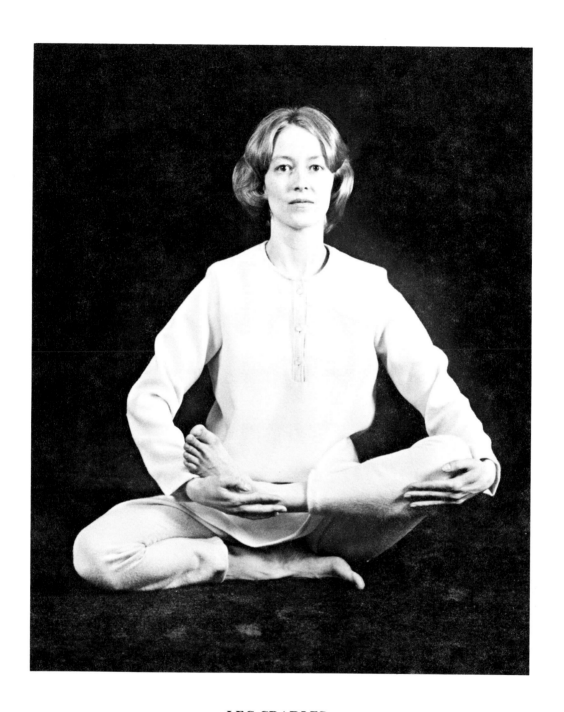

LEG CRADLES
FIRST POSITION

SECOND POSITION

Cradle the left leg by placing the foot in the bend of the right elbow and the knee in the bend of the left elbow. Interlace the fingers in front of the leg.

Gently rock the leg from side to side, gradually pulling it higher and closer to the body. Then hold both the knee and the foot to the chest for 5 seconds.

Relax and repeat with the right leg.

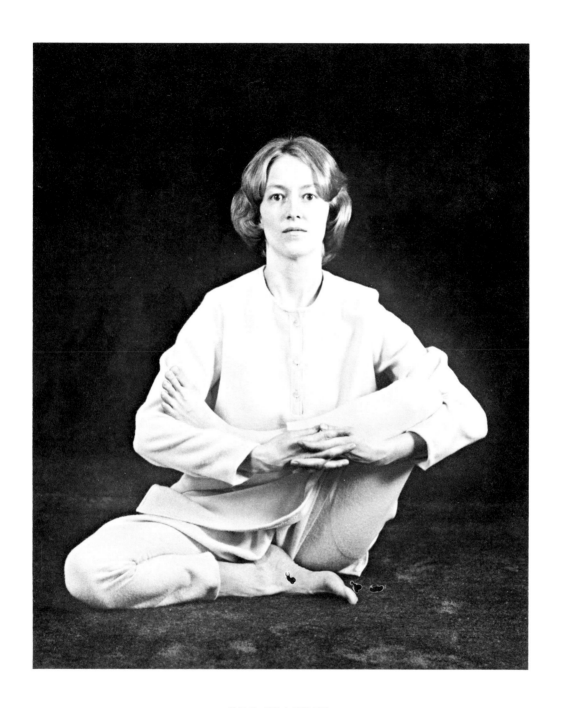

**LEG CRADLES
SECOND POSITION**

BUTTERFLY

Sit with the head, neck, and trunk straight, with the legs together and fully extended in front of you. Bend the knees, place the soles of the feet together, and bring the heels as close to the body as possible. Interlace the fingers and place them around the toes.

FIRST POSITION

Slowly and gently bounce the legs; try to lower the knees toward the floor. It is important to keep the movement of the legs gentle and relaxed. Do not try to force the knees to the floor.

SECOND POSITION

Rhythmically lower and raise the legs, coordinating the movements with the breath: exhale as you lower the knees toward the floor, and inhale as you raise the legs as high as possible.

Release the hands and extend the legs. With a gentle bouncing motion, alternate raising one knee while lowering the other in order to relax the muscles of the inner thighs.

THIRD POSITION

Return to the basic butterfly position, with the soles of the feet together, the heels as close to the body as possible, and the fingers interlaced around the toes.

Inhaling, expand the chest and stretch up from the base of the spine; extend the chin forward. Maintaining this stretch, exhale as you come forward as far as possible with the back straight. Then allow the head to relax downward toward the toes. Breathe evenly and hold to your comfortable capacity.

Inhaling, slowly raise the trunk.

Release the hands, extend the legs, and relax.

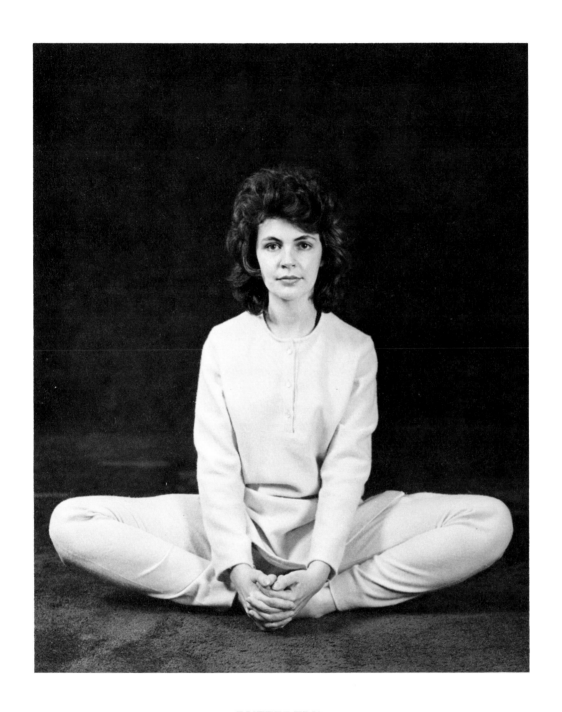

BUTTERFLY

LION (*Simhasana*)

This exercise involves the whole body, but focuses the attention on the mouth and throat.

Sit in the kneeling posture, *vajrasana* (see p. 89), with the top of the feet on the floor and the buttocks resting on the heels. Keep the head, neck, and trunk straight. Place the palms of the hands on the knees.

Exhaling, lift the body slightly off the heels and lean forward. In the same movement, straighten the arms, keeping the hands on the knees, and spread the fingers apart. Open the mouth as wide as possible and thrust the tongue out and down, trying to touch the chin. Gaze at the point between the two eyebrows. The whole body should feel tensed. Do not inhale while holding this position.

Then inhale, relax, and sit back on the heels.

Benefits:

- Makes the voice soft and melodious.
- Aids in relieving a sore throat.
- Is said to cure bad breath.

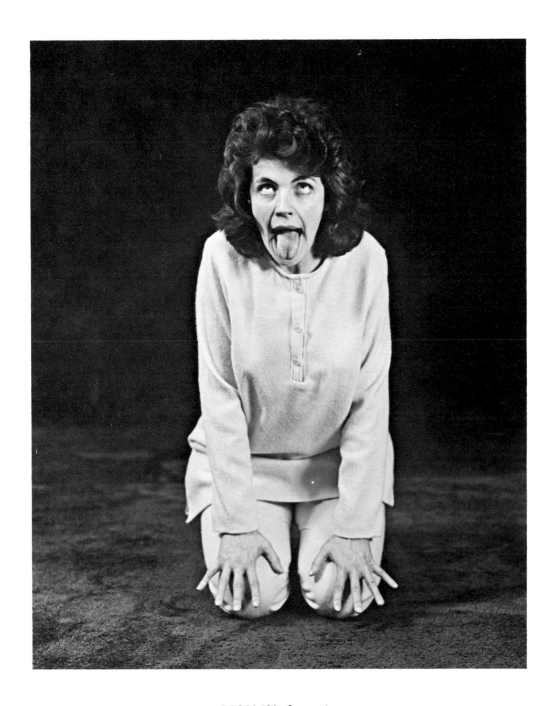

LION (*Simhasana*)

SYMBOL OF YOGA (*Yoga Mudra*)

Sit in the easy posture (see p. 88). Reach behind the back and grasp the right wrist with the left hand.

Exhaling, bend forward, keeping the back straight as long as possible. Slowly lower the body until the forehead rests on the floor in front of the legs. Keep the arms and hands relaxed and do not lift the buttocks off the floor.

Breathe evenly; hold 10 to 15 seconds.

Inhaling, slowly return to a sitting position, with the back straight. Release the hands, stretch the legs, and relax completely.

NOTE: This is a simplified version; in the full yoga mudra the student sits in the full lotus posture.

Variation: Sitting in the kneeling posture, *vajrasana* (see p. 89), place the fists on the abdomen at the inside of the hip bones, bend forward, and place the forehead on the floor.

Breathe evenly; hold 10 to 15 seconds.

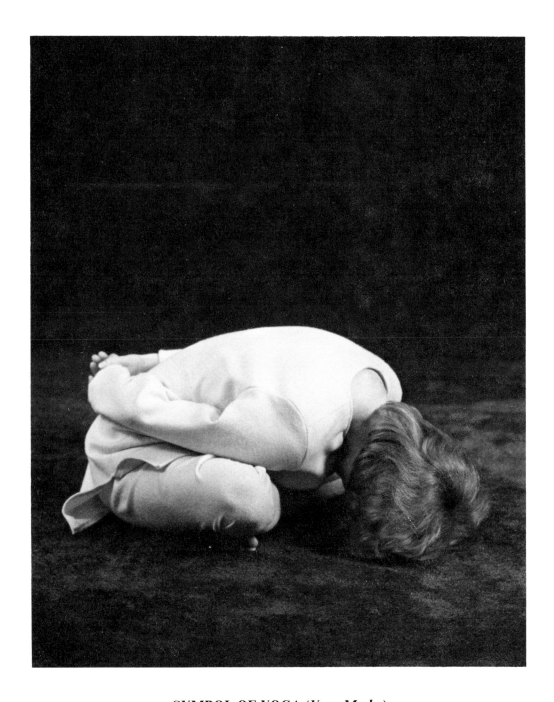

SYMBOL OF YOGA (*Yoga Mudra*)

SQUATTING POSTURE

FIRST VARIATION

Sit in a squatting position with the feet parallel and flat on the floor, 12 to 18 inches apart.

Allow the arms to rest over the knees and grasp the arms above the elbow with the hands.

SECOND VARIATION

Unlock the arms and shift the feet so that they are 8 to 12 inches apart.

Place the elbows on the knees, covering the face gently with the palms of the hands. Do not cover the nostrils or put pressure on the eyes.

Breathe evenly. To advance the posture, bring the feet closer together and gradually increase the time the posture is held.

NOTE: Persons with knee problems should exercise caution in performing this posture.

Benefits:

- Especially useful for relieving dizziness and stomach cramps.
- Develops balance.
- Stretches the muscles on the front side of the thighs.
- Helps in elimination; stimulates the peristaltic movement of materials through the digestive tract.
- Relieves aching of the ankles and knees.

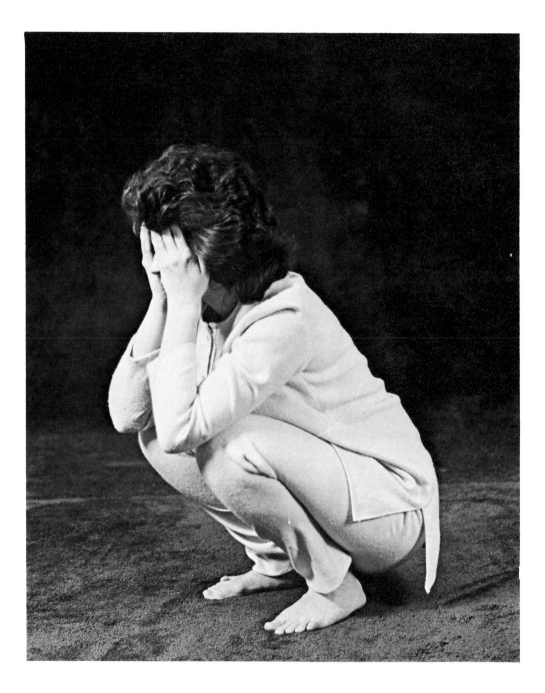

**SQUATTING POSTURE
SECOND VARIATION**

COW'S FACE (*Gomukhasana*)

FIRST STEP

Sit with the head, neck, and trunk straight, with the legs together and fully extended in front of you.

Bend the left leg and place the heel next to the right hip.

Bend the right knee, crossing the right leg over the left, and place the heel of the right leg next to the left hip. The knees are aligned (the right knee on top of the left), and the buttocks remain firmly on the floor.

Place the hands on the soles of the feet. (Alternatively, you may place the left hand on the right knee and the right hand on top of the left hand, or you may interlace the fingers and rest the palms of the hands on the right knee or between the knees.)

Repeat the posture, reversing the position of the legs.

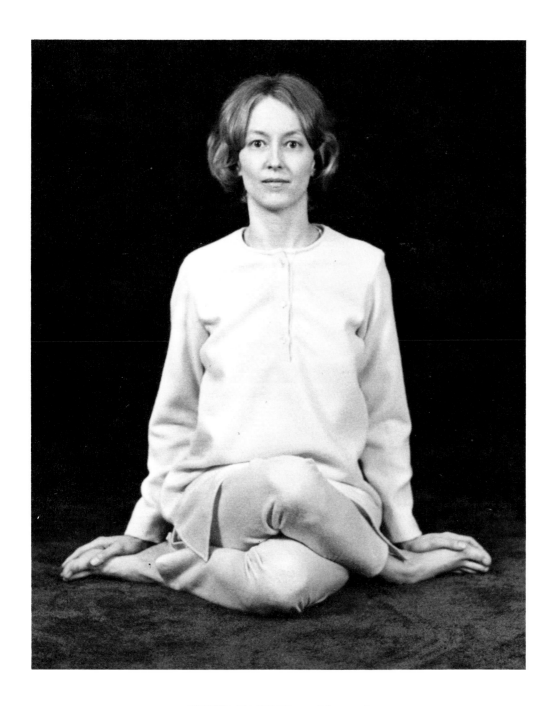

COW'S FACE (*Gomukhasana*)
FIRST STEP

SECOND STEP

Raise the right arm overhead, bending it at the elbow, and place the right palm between the shoulder blades. Lower the left arm behind the back, bending it at the elbow, with the palm facing outward. Clasp the fingers of both hands together. The right elbow points toward the ceiling and the left elbow toward the floor. Breathe evenly; hold for 15 seconds, stretching the arms, shoulders, and chest.

Repeat the posture, reversing the position of the legs and hands.

NOTE: If you cannot clasp your hands, you may grasp a handkerchief or some other type of cloth between the hands, using the cloth to slowly bring the hands together.

Benefits:

- Is said to remove rheumatism in the legs and to cure hemorrhoids.

- Is especially good for learning to breathe diaphragmatically, since the relative immobilization of the thorax and shoulders makes thoracic breathing inconvenient.

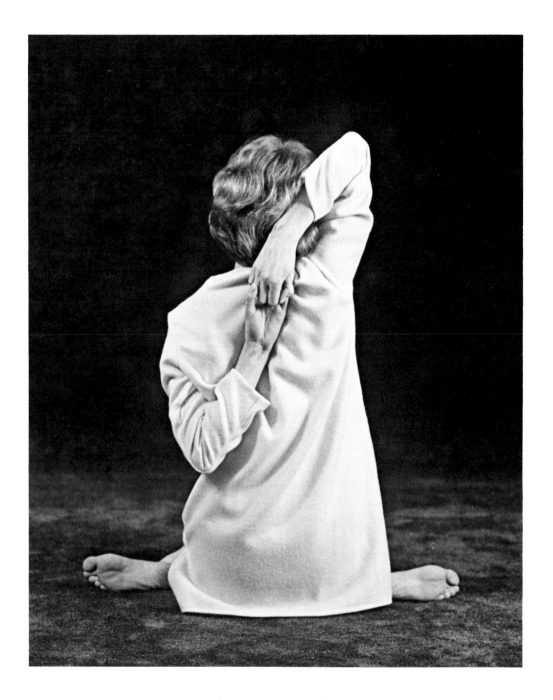

COW'S FACE (*Gomukhasana*)
SECOND STEP

C. BACKWARD-BENDING POSTURES

COBRA (*Bhujangasana*)

Lie on the stomach, with the forehead resting on the floor, legs and feet together, with the body fully extended and relaxed. Bend the elbows, keeping them close to the body, and place the hands palms down beside the chest, aligning the fingertips with the nipples.

Inhaling, slowly begin to raise the head, allowing first the nose and then the chin to touch the floor as the head is stretched forward and upward. Without using the strength of the arms or hands, slowly raise the shoulders and chest; look up and bend back as far as possible. Breathe evenly; hold for 5 seconds.

Exhaling, slowly lower the body until the forehead rests on the floor. Relax.

In this posture the navel remains on the floor. To lift the thorax, use the muscles of the back only. Do not use the arms and hands to push the body off the floor, but to balance the body. Keep the feet and legs together and relaxed.

NOTE: There are many variations of this posture. One common variation entails using the arms to raise the thorax. We do not recommend this variation for beginners, as it makes it easy for one to force the body beyond its capacity.

Benefits:

- Strengthens the muscles of the shoulders, neck, and back.

- Develops flexibility of the cervical vertebrae.

- Corrects deviations of the spine.

- Improves circulation to the intervertebral discs.

- Expands the chest and develops elasticity of the lungs.

- Is said to help low back pain, constipation, gastric pains, gas pains, and backaches.

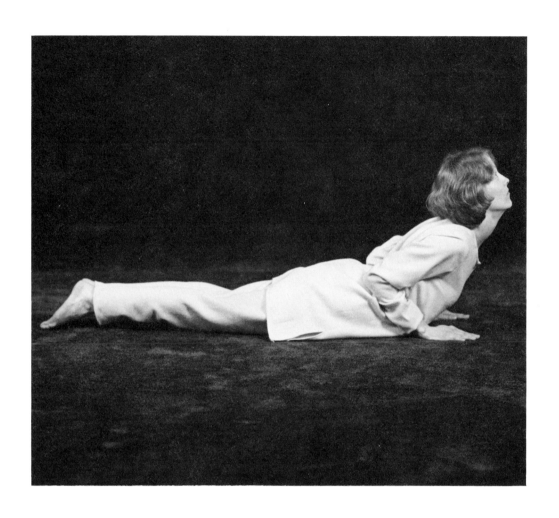

COBRA (*Bhujangasana*)

HORSE MUDRA (*Ashvini Mudra*)

Lie in the crocodile posture (see p. 16), but with the legs together. Slowly, in a rolling motion, pull the buttocks inward. Contract the anal sphincter muscles and pull the anus inward and upward. Hold for 2 to 3 seconds. Relax. Repeat 7 to 10 times. After this exercise is mastered in a lying position, it can also be practiced in a standing position.

Benefits:

- Tones the buttocks and the anal sphincter muscles.

- Can be helpful for people suffering from constipation or hemorrhoids.

- Is a good preparation for *mulabandha,* the root lock used in pranayama exercises and meditation.

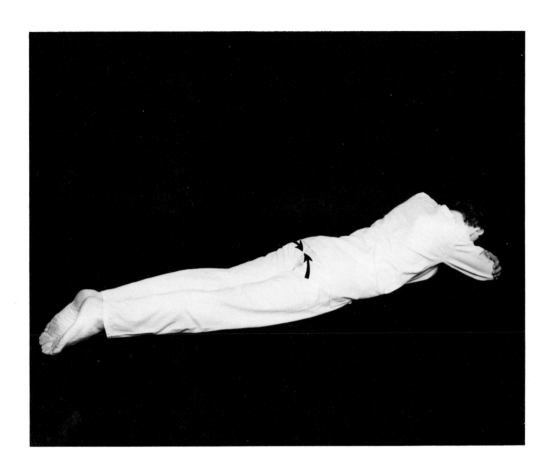

HORSE MUDRA (*Ashvini Mudra*)

Arrows show direction of muscular contraction.

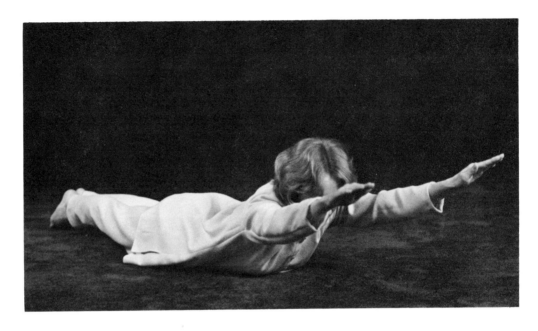

HALF BOAT (*Ardha Naukasana*)

VARIATION 1

Lie on the stomach with the forehead on the floor and the arms extended straight overhead with the palms resting on the floor. Keep the feet and legs together and relaxed.

Inhaling, raise the chest, arms, and head from the floor while keeping the head between the arms. Breathe evenly; hold for 5 seconds.

Exhaling, lower the body. Relax.

NOTE: Both variations of the half boat should be practiced for at least one week before attempting the full boat posture.

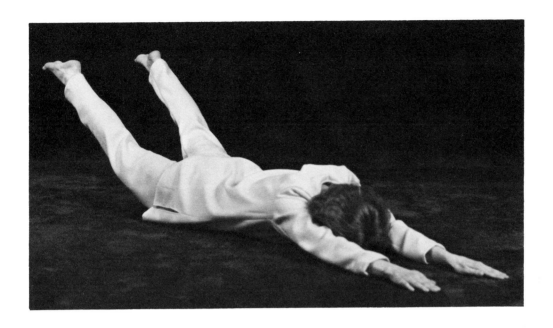

HALF BOAT (*Ardha Naukasana*)

VARIATION 2

Lie on the stomach with the forehead on the floor and the arms extended straight overhead with the palms resting on the floor. Keep the hands, arms, and chest relaxed; keep the legs straight and the feet approximately 12 to 18 inches apart.

Inhaling, raise the legs and feet from the floor. Breathe evenly; hold for 5 seconds.

Exhaling, lower the legs. Relax.

BOAT (*Naukasana*)

The boat posture combines the two variations of the half boat. Lie on the stomach with the forehead on the floor and the arms extended straight overhead with the palms resting on the floor. Keep the hands, arms, and chest relaxed; keep the legs straight and the feet approximately 18 inches apart.

Inhaling, simultaneously raise the arms and the legs until only the abdomen remains on the floor. The body forms a gentle curve from the tips of the toes to the tips of the fingers. Breathe evenly; hold for 5 seconds.

Exhaling, lower the body. Relax.

NOTE: For a greater stretch, with the head between the arms try to look up at the ceiling. Also, as the body becomes stronger, the legs can be brought close together.

Benefits:

- Strengthens all the muscles of the back.

- Increases intra-abdominal pressure and promotes better circulation to the internal organs.

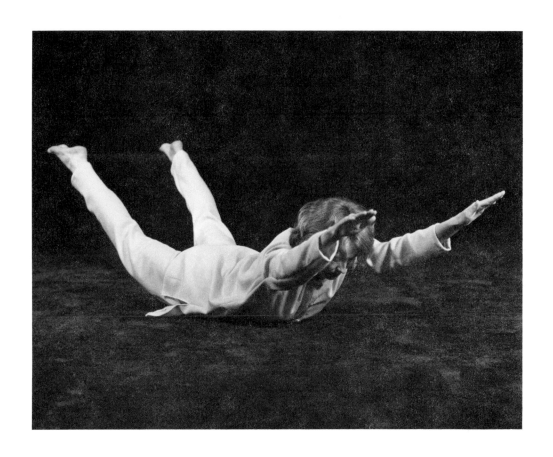

BOAT (*Naukasana*)

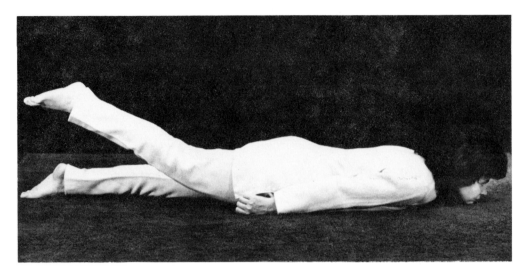

HALF LOCUST (*Ardha Shalabhasana*)

Lie on the stomach with the legs together and the arms extended along the sides of the body; place the chin on the floor. Make fists with the hands, placing the thumbs and forefingers on the floor.

Inhaling, and without bending the knee or twisting the body sideways, raise the right leg as high as possible. The pelvic bones should remain on the floor. The left leg remains relaxed; do not allow the left knee to press against the floor.

Breathe evenly. Hold for 5 seconds.

Exhaling, slowly lower the leg.

Repeat with the left leg. Then, continuing to alternate legs, perform the exercise twice more with each leg.

Variation: Lie in the beginning position described above. Inhaling, raise the right leg only 4 inches above the floor; then stretch the leg from the hip through the toes. Breathe evenly and hold for 5 seconds.

Maintaining the leg 4 inches above the floor, move it 30° to the side. Breathe evenly and hold for 5 seconds, keeping the leg stretched from the hip through the toes.

Exhaling, relax the stretch in the leg, take it back to the starting position, and slowly lower.

Repeat with the left leg.

NOTE: Practice the half locust for at least two weeks, slowly increasing the time held to 10 seconds, before attempting the full locust.

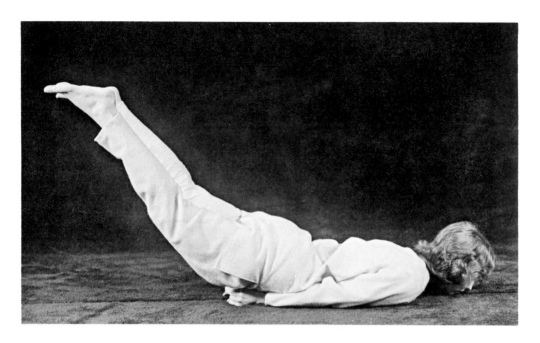

LOCUST (*Shalabhasana*)

Assume the position described at the start of the half locust. Keeping the arms straight, place the fists under the top of the thighs.

Inhaling, raise both legs as high as possible. Breathe evenly; hold for 5 seconds.

Exhaling, slowly lower the legs and relax.

NOTE: For beginning students the fists should remain under the thighs. This enables one to raise the legs and feet higher in the air. As the abdominal muscles and the muscles of the back become stronger, the fists can be placed at the sides of the body.

Benefits:

- Strengthens the muscles of the lower back, thus improving sitting postures for meditation.

- Reduces lower back pain tendencies.

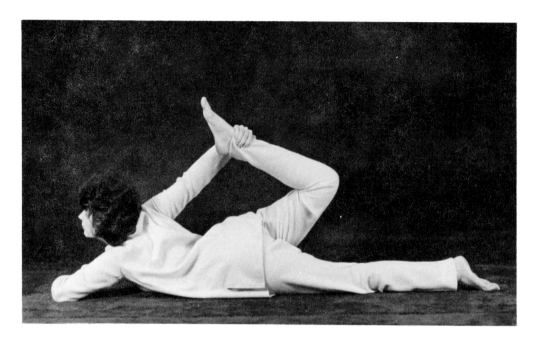

HALF BOW (*Ardha Dhanurasana*)

VARIATION 1

Lie on the stomach with the legs together, the chin on the floor, the right arm extended alongside the body, and the left arm bent at the elbow and placed on the floor in front of the head.

Bend the right leg at the knee, and with the right hand grasp the outside of the ankle. Inhaling, raise the head, shoulders, and chest, pulling the leg up as far as possible without straining the muscles of the back. Breathe evenly; hold for 5 seconds.

Exhaling, slowly lower the leg and then the rest of the body.

Relax.

Repeat the exercise on the left side.

Alternating sides, repeat the exercise one or two more times with each leg.

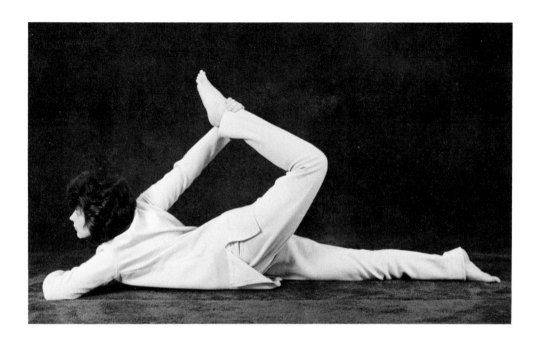

HALF BOW (*Ardha Dhanurasana*)

VARIATION 2

Lie in the position described at the start of Variation 1.

Bend the left leg at the knee. This time grasp the inside of the left ankle with the right hand.

Inhaling, raise the head, shoulders, and chest, pulling the leg up as far as possible. Breathe evenly; hold for 5 seconds.

Exhaling, slowly lower the leg and then the rest of the body.

Relax.

Repeat the exercise on the right side.

Alternating sides, repeat the exercise one or two more times with each leg.

BOW (*Dhanurasana*)

Lie on the stomach with the arms extended alongside the body. Place the chin on the floor.

Bend both legs at the knees. Keeping the arms on the outside of the legs, grasp the ankles.

Inhaling, raise the head, shoulders, and chest; then pull the legs up as high as possible. The body should resemble the smooth curve of a bow. Breathe evenly; hold for 5 seconds.

Exhaling, slowly lower the legs until the knees are on the floor; then lower the torso. Relax.

Repeat the exercise one or two more times.

NOTE: Beginners should allow the legs to be apart. In this exercise the strength of the arms is being used to further the suppleness of the back, and due caution should be taken not to strain.

Benefits:

- Develops flexibility of the spine.
- Stretches the abdominal muscles and massages them.
- Prepares you for more difficult backward-bending postures, such as the wheel and the scorpion.
- Reduces fat.
- Strengthens the knee joints.

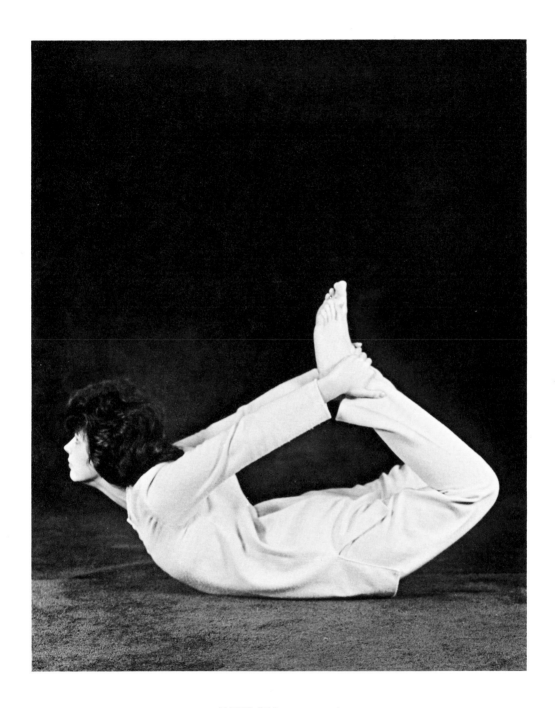

BOW (*Dhanurasana*)

D. FORWARD-BENDING POSTURES

PREPARATION FOR HEAD-TO-KNEE POSTURE AND POSTERIOR STRETCH

Sit with the head, neck, and trunk straight and the legs extended in front of you as far apart as possible.

A. Inhaling, raise the arms overhead, stretch up, and expand the chest. Exhaling, with the back straight and the head between the arms, bend forward and place the hands as close to the right foot as possible. Breathe evenly and hold for 5 seconds. Be sure that the backs of the knees remain on the floor.

Inhaling, and keeping the arms next to the head, slowly return to a sitting position.

B. Repeat, bending toward the left leg.

C. Repeat, bending straight forward between the legs.

D. Repeat, with the soles of the feet together and the heels as close to the body as possible (as in the butterfly [see p. 96]).

This series can be repeated until the body feels limber enough to practice the head-to-knee posture and the posterior stretch. The length of time each position is held can be varied.

HEAD-TO-KNEE POSTURE
(*Janushirshasana*)

Sit with the head, neck, and trunk straight and the legs together, extended in front of the body. Bend the right leg at the knee and place the sole of the right foot on the inside of the left thigh. Position the heel snugly against the perineum.

Inhaling, raise the arms overhead, stretch up, and expand the chest. Exhaling, with the back straight and the head between the arms, bend forward as far as possible, placing the hands comfortably on the left leg. The back of the left knee should remain on the floor. Relax, breathe evenly and hold for 5 to 10 seconds.

To further the stretch: remain in position; inhale and stretch forward from the base of the spine to the crown of the head. Exhaling, bring the head further down toward the left leg. Relax and breathe evenly.

Inhaling, and keeping the arms next to the head, slowly stretch up and return to a sitting position.

Exhaling, lower the arms and relax.

Repeat with the right leg extended and the left knee bent.

Advanced Variation: Follow the instructions as described above, but this time grasp the big toe of the extended leg with both hands. Bring the head to the knee and place the elbows on either side of the knee.

Repeat on the opposite side.

Benefits:

- Useful for treating disorders of the prostate gland.

- Helpful for men in controlling sexual urges because of the gentle pressure on the prostate gland.

126

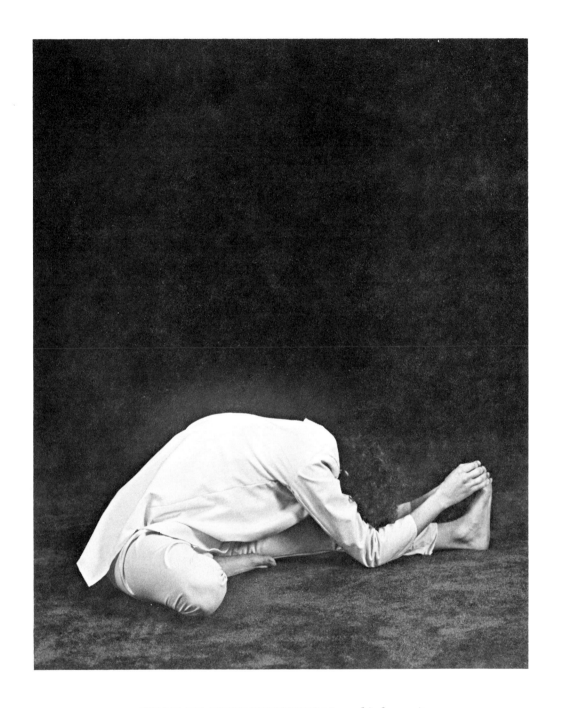

HEAD-TO-KNEE POSTURE (*Janushirshasana*)
ADVANCED VARIATION

POSTERIOR STRETCH
(*Paschimottanasana*)

Sit with the head, neck, and trunk straight and the legs together, extended in front of the body. Inhaling, raise the arms overhead, stretch up, and expand the chest. Exhaling, with the back straight and the head between the arms, bend forward as far as possible, placing the hands comfortably on the legs. The backs of the knees should remain on the floor. Relax, breathe evenly, and hold for 5 to 10 seconds.

To further the stretch: Remain in position; inhale and stretch forward from the base of the spine to the crown of the head. Exhaling, bring the head further down toward the legs. Relax and breathe evenly.

Advanced Variation: Grasp your two big toes with your thumbs and index fingers. Bring the head to the knees and place the elbows on the floor next to the knees. Breathe evenly; hold for 5 to 10 seconds.

Benefits:

- Stimulates the peristaltic movement of materials through the digestive tract and prevents constipation.

- Stimulates the entire abdominal area: kidneys, liver, stomach, spleen, pancreas.

- Cures indigestion and poor appetite.

- Is said to ameliorate diabetes.

- Stretches the hamstring muscles of the thighs and the muscles and ligaments of the back, and is thus a good preparation for the sitting postures of meditation.

- Gently massages the intervertebral discs, aids in their circulation, and develops flexibility of the spinal column.

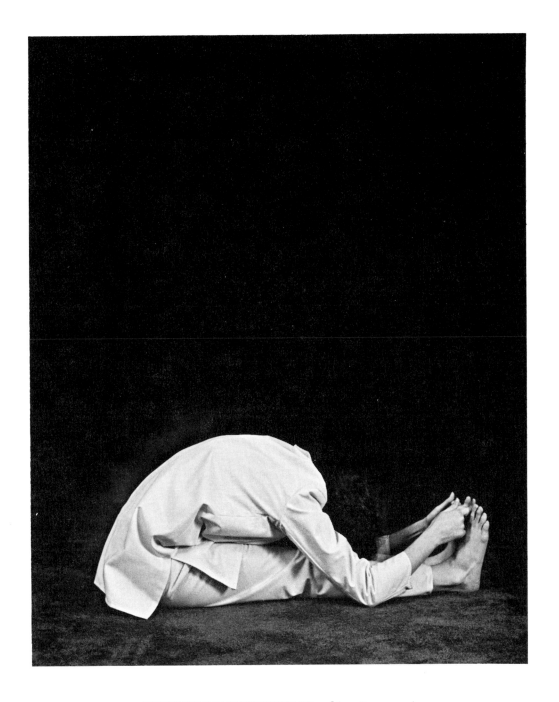

POSTERIOR STRETCH (*Paschimottanasana*)
ADVANCED VARIATION

129

INCLINED PLANE (*Katikasana*)

Sit on the floor with the head, neck, and trunk straight and with the legs together, extended in front of the body. Leaning back slightly, place the hands on the floor 8 to 10 inches behind the hips, pointing the fingers away from the body.

Inhaling, raise the entire body until it forms an inclined plane from the shoulders to the toes. The bottom of the feet press against the floor, the arms remain straight, and the head drops back as far as possible.

Breathe evenly; hold for 5 seconds.

Exhaling, slowly lower the body and return to a sitting position.

Benefits:

- Exercises the back muscles.

- Complements the stretch of the forward-bending postures.

- Firms hips, abdomen, thighs, and arms.

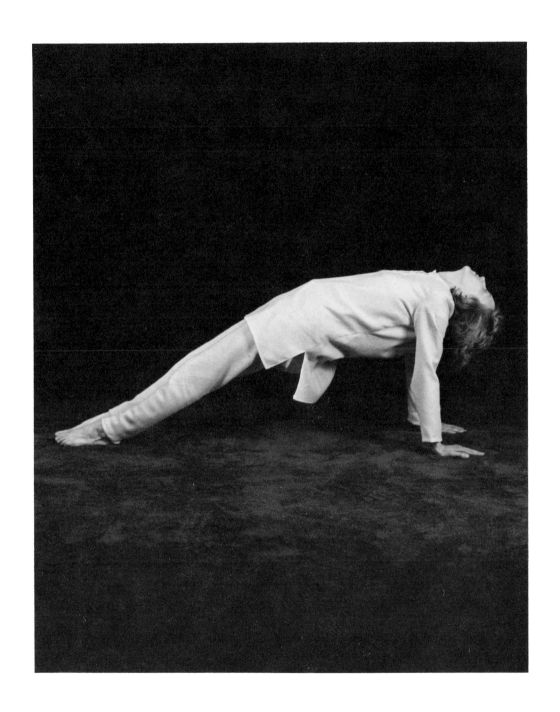

INCLINED PLANE (*Katikasana*)

E. TWISTING POSTURES

TWISTING POSTURE

This is a preparatory exercise for the spinal twist.

Lie on the back with the legs together and extended on the floor, and the arms extended at shoulder level with the palms on the floor.

Inhaling, bend the knees and draw them to the chest.

Exhaling, slowly bring the knees to the floor near the right elbow and at the same time twist the head to the left. Keep the shoulders and arms firmly on the floor. Breathe evenly; hold for 5 seconds.

Inhaling, bring the knees back to the chest and the head back to the center.

Exhaling, repeat on the opposite side, bringing the knees to the floor near the left elbow and turning the head to the right. Breathe evenly; hold for 5 seconds.

Alternating sides, repeat the exercise two more times on each side. Then, having brought the knees back to the chest and the head back to the center, exhale and slowly lower the legs to the floor; relax.

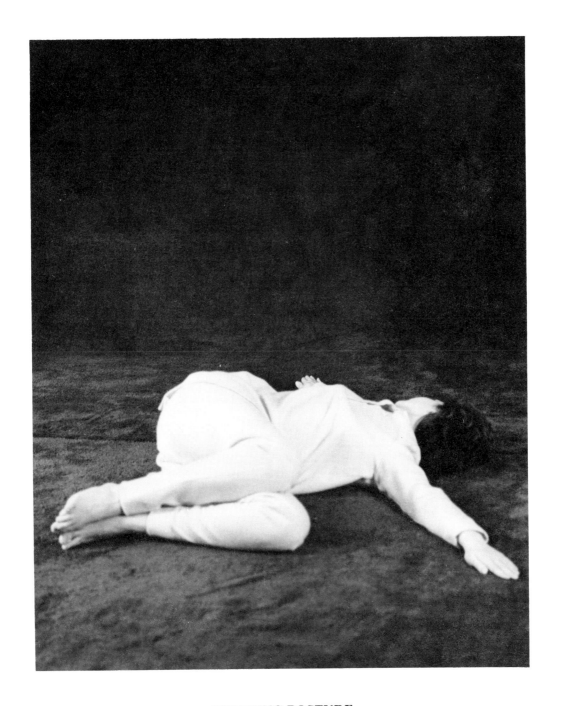

TWISTING POSTURE

HALF SPINAL TWIST
(*Ardha Matsyendrasana*)

Sit with the head, neck, and trunk straight and with the legs together, extended in front of the body.

Bend the left leg and place the left foot on the floor at the outside of the right knee. Twist the body toward the left and place the left hand approximately 4 to 6 inches behind the left hip, fingers pointing away from the body. Bring the right arm over the outside of the left leg and grasp the left foot with the right hand.

When bringing the arm over the leg, you may bend slightly forward if necessary; however, do not arch back and then twist the body.

Keeping the back straight, turn to the left, twisting from the lower spine, and look over the left shoulder. Do not use the arms to force the body further into the twist, but use the arms for balance only.

Breathe evenly; hold for 5 seconds.

Repeat on the opposite side.

Benefits:

- Provides twist to the spinal column, stretching and lengthening the muscles and ligaments and keeping the spine elastic and healthy.

- Alternately compresses each half of the abdominal region, squeezing the internal organs and promoting better circulation through them.

- Combats constipation, reduces fat, and improves digestion.

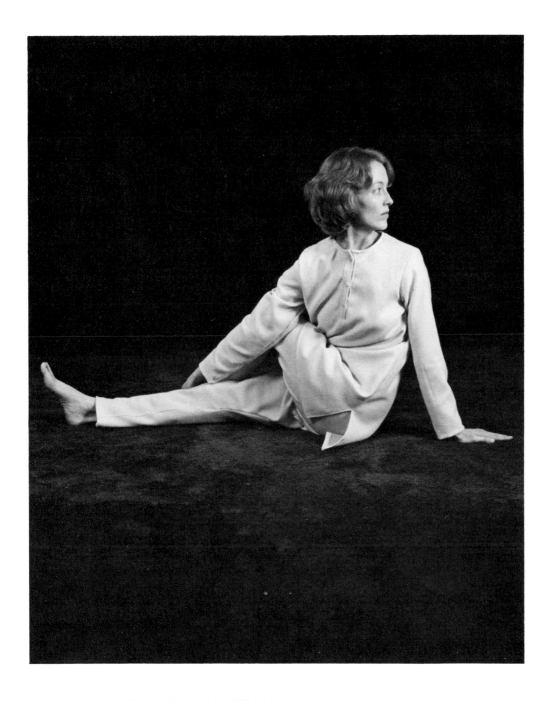

HALF SPINAL TWIST (*Ardha Matsyendrasana*)

F. LEG LIFTS

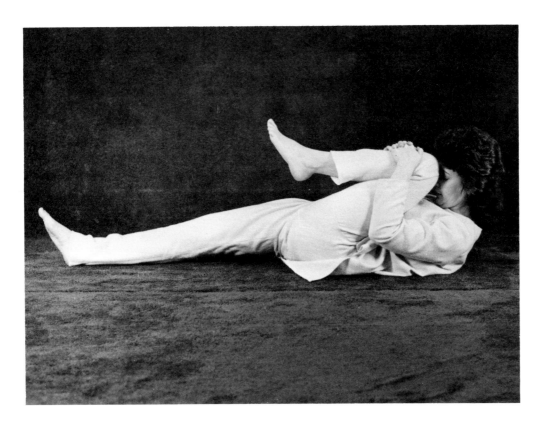

WIND-ELIMINATING POSTURE
(*Pavanamuktasana*)

Lie on the back and breathe evenly. Bend the right knee, wrap the arms around the leg, and pull the leg toward the chest. Raise the head and bring the forehead toward the knee. Breathe evenly and hold for 3 to 5 seconds.

Lower the leg to the floor and relax.

Repeat with the left leg.

Then repeat with both legs at once.

Benefits:

- Relieves gas in the lower digestive tract.

SINGLE LEG LIFTS
(*Utthita Ekapadasana*)

Lie on the back with the legs together, flat on the floor. Place the arms along the sides of the body with the palms on the floor.

Inhaling, slowly raise the right leg as high as possible. Keep both legs straight.

Breathe evenly; hold for 5 seconds. Exhaling, slowly lower the leg.

Repeat with the left leg. Then, continuing to alternate legs, repeat the exercise two more times with each leg.

NOTE: Throughout the exercise, keep the shoulders, arms, and hands relaxed. While lifting the leg, do not press the arms against the floor, nor twist the body to the side. While raising one leg, keep the opposite leg straight, resting it firmly on the floor. If in the beginning you find this difficult, bend the opposite leg at the knee and place the foot on the floor. Practice in this manner until the abdominal and lower back muscles are strengthened; then the exercise can be practiced with the legs straight.

Variation 1: Repeat the exercise as described above, but raise the leg only 4 inches from the floor.

Variation 2: Repeat the exercise as described above, but raise the leg at a 45° angle from the floor.

Variation 3: After raising the leg perpendicular to the floor, point the toe toward the ceiling and hold for 3 seconds. Then push the heel toward the ceiling and again hold for 3 seconds. Relax the foot and slowly lower the leg. Alternating legs, repeat two more times with each leg.

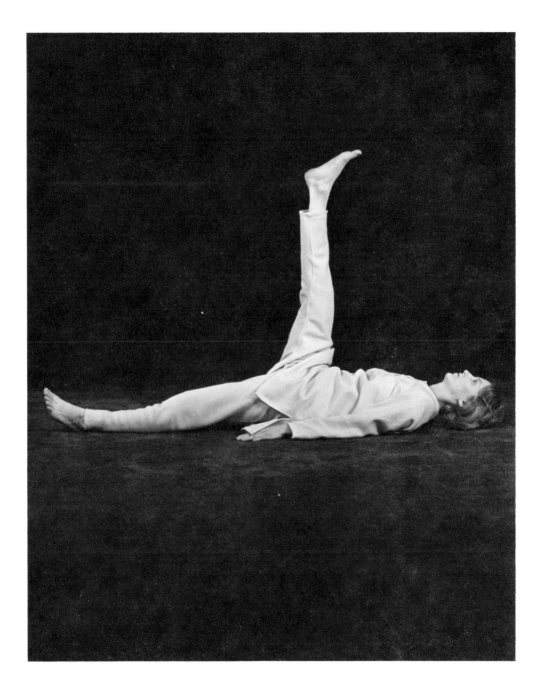

SINGLE LEG LIFTS (*Utthita Ekapadasana*)

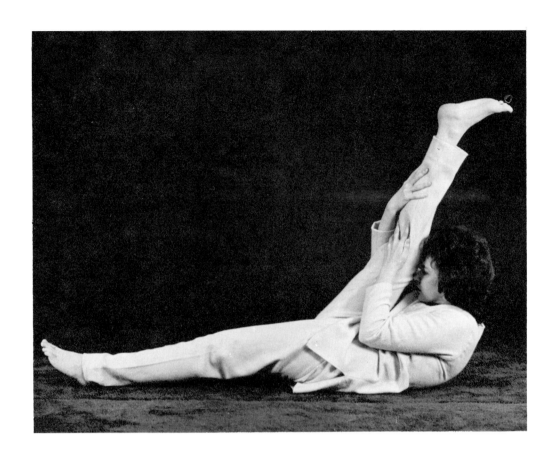

SINGLE LEG LIFTS (*Utthita Ekapadasana*)

Variation 4: After raising the leg, grasp the calf or, if possible, the ankle. Pull the leg toward the head; raising the shoulders from the floor, try to touch the head to the knee. Breathe evenly; hold for 3 seconds.

Exhaling, relax and slowly lower the leg. Repeat with the other leg.

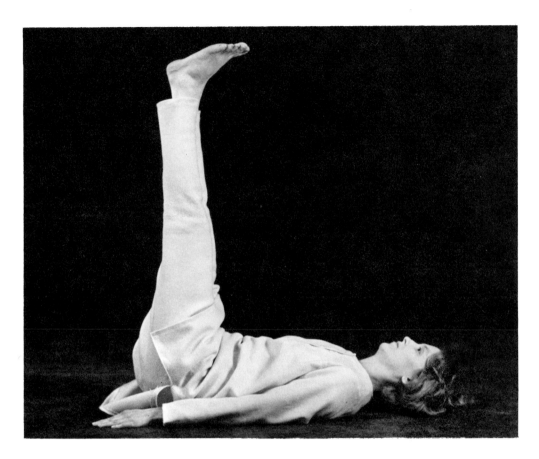

DOUBLE LEG LIFTS
(*Utthita Dvipadasana*)

Lie on the back with the legs together, flat on the floor. Place the arms along the sides of the body with the palms on the floor. Inhaling, raise both legs—keeping them straight—until they are perpendicular to the floor. Breathe evenly; hold for 5 seconds.

Exhaling, slowly lower the legs.

NOTE: If in the beginning you find that keeping the legs straight is too difficult, you may instead bend the knees and bring them to the chest. Then place the hands under the hips, straighten the legs, and slowly lower.

Variations: Perform with both legs the four variations of the single leg lifts described on pp. 140 and 142.

BALANCE ON HIPS
(*Utthita Hastapadasana*)

Lie on the back with the legs together and flat on the floor and the arms alongside the body with the palms on the floor. Stretching the hands toward the toes and keeping the arms and legs straight, raise both the trunk and the legs until only the hips remain on the floor. Hold for 5 seconds. Lower and relax.

The balance on hips posture is sometimes referred to as the boat posture.

Benefits:

- Excellent for developing balance and strengthening the abdominal muscles.

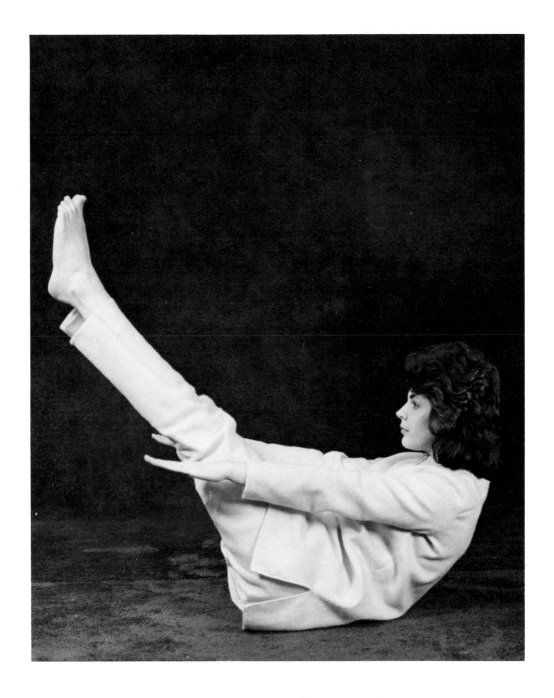

BALANCE ON HIPS (*Utthita Hastapadasana*)

G. INVERTED POSTURES

ROCKING CHAIR

This is a preparatory exercise for the plow posture.

Variation 1

Sitting on the floor, bend the knees and bring them toward the chest; do not cross the legs. Interlace the fingers and place them on the backs of the thighs just above the knees. Round the back and tuck the head in toward the knees. Slowly rock back onto the shoulders; then rock forward, returning to the starting position.

Using momentum to rock gently back and forth, try to be aware of each vertebra as it touches the floor. Do not hold either the forward or the backward position. Rock back and forth five times.

Variation 2

Sitting on the floor, bend the knees, bringing them up to the chest, and cross the legs at the ankles. With the arms on the outside of the legs, grasp the toes.

Keeping the head tucked in toward the legs, rock backward as if in a backward somersault, and touch the toes to the floor behind the head. Then rock forward in the same way until the forehead touches the floor between the knees. Do not lift the hips off the floor when attempting to bring the forehead to the floor.

Using momentum to rock gently back and forth, perform the exercise five times.

Benefits:

- Limbers the vertebrae and stretches the muscles of the back, and thus is a good warm-up exercise for the forward-bending and backward-bending postures.

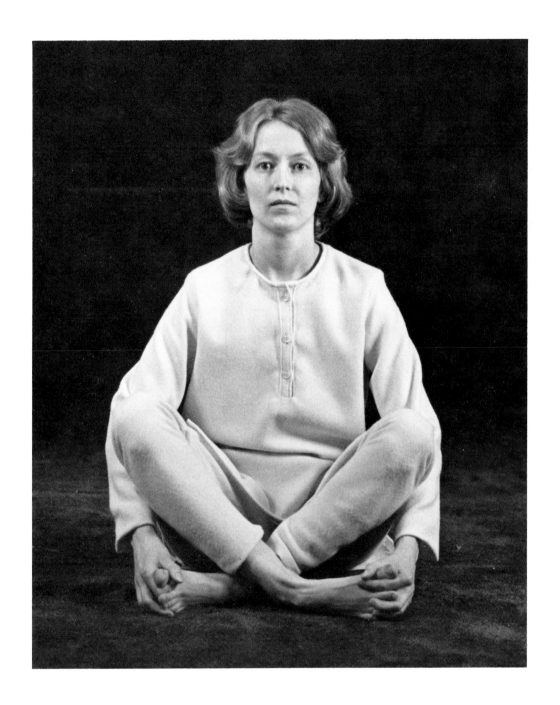

**ROCKING CHAIR
VARIATION 2**

HALF PLOW (*Ardha Halasana*)

Lie on the back with the legs together and flat on the floor and the arms alongside the body with the palms on the floor.

Inhaling, slowly raise both legs until they are perpendicular to the floor. Then raise the hips off the floor, keeping the legs straight and together. Extend the feet beyond the head until the legs are parallel to the floor. Breathe evenly; hold for 10 to 15 seconds.

Exhaling, slowly lower the hips and return the legs to a perpendicular position. Continue exhaling and slowly lower the legs to the floor.

NOTE: Beginning students can support the back by bending the arms and placing the hands on the hips. Also, to come out of the posture smoothly, it may be helpful to raise the chin slightly so that the head does not come off the floor.

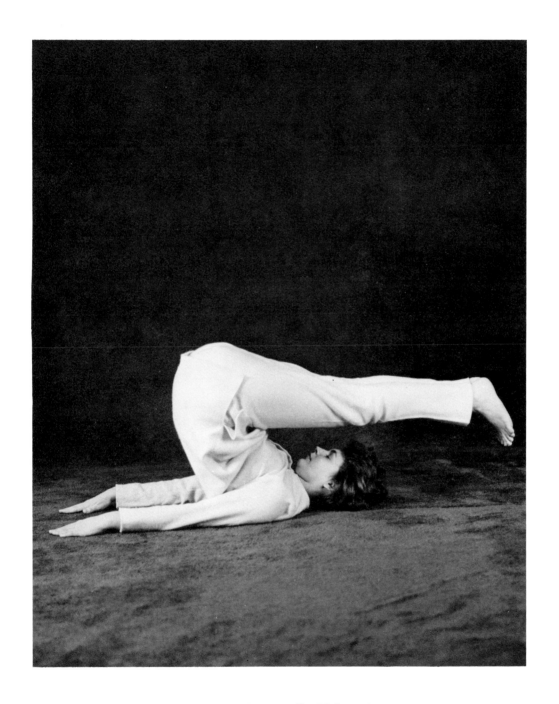

HALF PLOW (*Ardha Halasana*)

151

PLOW (*Halasana*)

Follow the instructions for the half plow (see p. 150) but continue to lower the feet until the toes touch the floor behind the head. Breathe evenly; hold for 15 to 20 seconds.

Exhaling, slowly lower the hips and return the legs to a perpendicular position. Continue exhaling and slowly lower the legs to the floor.

Slowly increase your capacity until you can hold the plow comfortably for one minute.

Benefits:

- Lengthens the muscles of the backs of the thighs and prepares the body for forward-bending and sitting postures.

- Relaxes the muscles of the back and gently stretches the ligaments of the spinal column.

- Is one of the most reviving and rejuvenating of all postures.

- Massages, tones, and stimulates all internal organs, especially the intestines, spleen, and liver.

- Is beneficial for constipation.

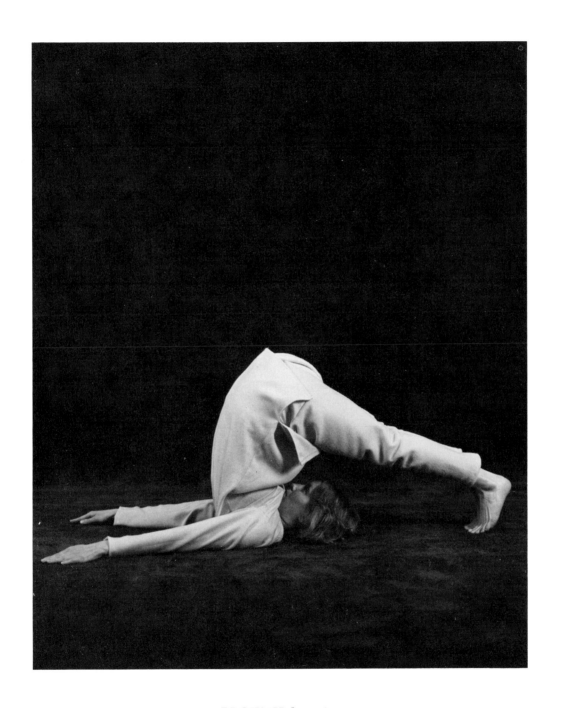

PLOW (*Halasana*)

INVERTED ACTION POSTURE
(*Viparitakarani*)

Assume the half plow posture (see p. 150).

Place the hands on the hips on either side of the spine, with the elbows a shoulders' width apart. Inhaling, raise both legs until they are perpendicular to the floor.

Breathe evenly; hold for 20 to 30 seconds.

Exhaling, slowly return to the half plow pose. Then lower the hips and return the legs to a perpendicular position. Continue exhaling and slowly lower the legs to the floor.

Slowly increase your capacity until you can hold the inverted action posture comfortably for one minute.

Benefits:

- Drains blood from the legs into the body cavities, relieving varicose veins.

- Diaphragmatic breathing can be learned effectively in this posture, due to the weight of the abdominal organs on the diaphragm.

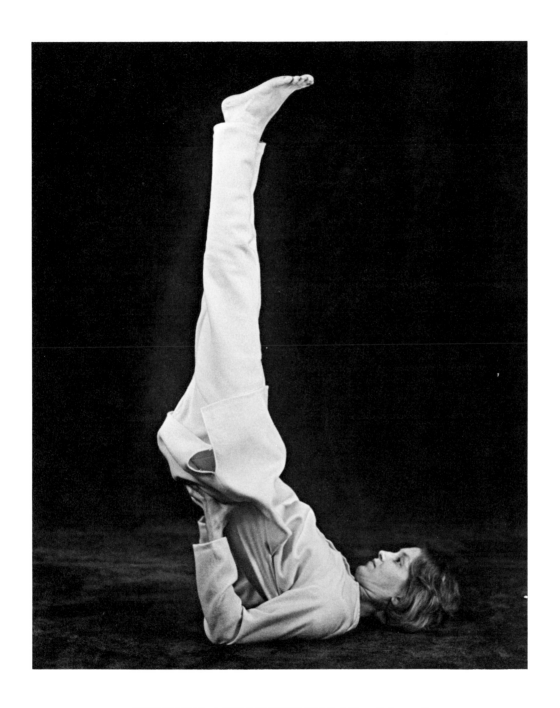

INVERTED ACTION POSTURE (*Viparitakarani*)

SHOULDERSTAND (*Sarvangasana*)

Assume the plow posture (see p. 152).

Bend the elbows and place the hands as close to the shoulders as possible, with the fingers pointing toward the small of the back and the elbows firmly on the floor. Raise both legs until they are perpendicular to the floor, lifting the hips toward the ceiling. Press the breastbone against the chin, gently at first and more firmly with experience. Keep the legs straight, relaxed, and perpendicular to the floor. Breathe evenly; hold for 20 to 30 seconds.

Slowly increase your capacity until you can hold this posture comfortably for one minute.

Benefits:

- As implied in the literal translation of *sarvangasana,* "all-members posture" or "entire-body posture," this posture benefits all parts of the body—the shoulders, arms, legs, head, neck, back, and internal organs.

- Strengthens arms, chest, and shoulders.

- Slims legs and hips.

- Strengthens the back and abdominal muscles.

- Places gentle traction on the cervical vertebrae, keeping this important area healthy and flexible.

- Venous drainage of the legs occurs quickly and completely, especially benefiting those persons with varicose veins.

- As in the inverted action posture, diaphragmatic breathing is easily observed and learned.

- Causes higher blood pressure and simple mechanical pressure in the neck, which are said to rejuvenate the thyroid and parathyroid glands, making them function optimally. These important glands regulate body weight and metabolism by natural mechanisms.

- Reduces the occurrence of acute and chronic throat ailments.

- Increases the blood supply to all the important structures of the neck.

- Called "the Queen of Asanas" and considered a panacea for internal organ ailments, especially those of old age, the shoulderstand combats indigestion, constipation, degeneration of the endocrine glands, and problems occurring in the liver, the gall bladder, the kidney, the pancreas, the spleen, and the digestive system.

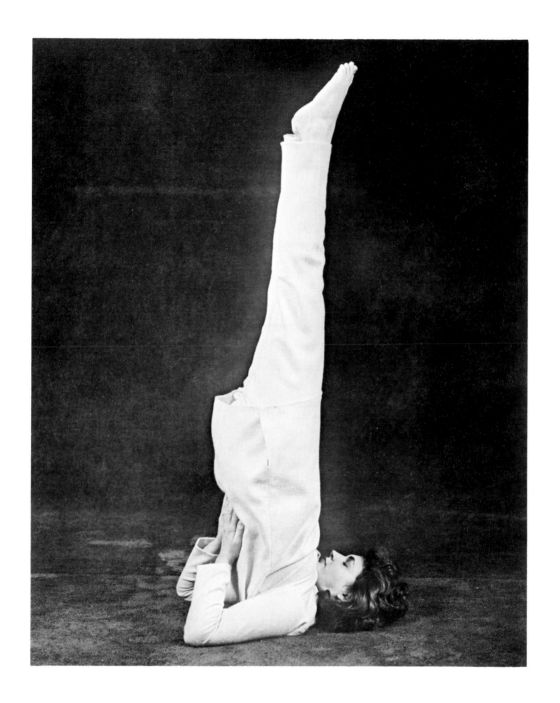

SHOULDERSTAND (*Sarvangasana*)

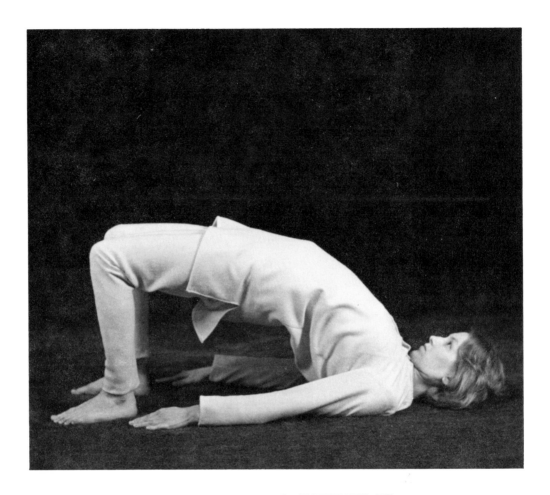

ARCH POSTURE

This is a preparatory exercise for the bridge posture.

Lie on the back and place the arms along the sides of the body with the palms downward. Bend the knees and bring the heels close to the buttocks.

Inhaling, raise the hips, abdomen, and chest off the floor as high as possible, arching the back, keeping the arms and hands on the floor and the legs close to each other.

Breathe evenly; hold for 5 seconds.

Exhaling, slowly lower the back to the floor and then extend the legs. Relax.

NOTE: When using this exercise to relax the back after the shoulderstand, beginners may support the back with the hands.

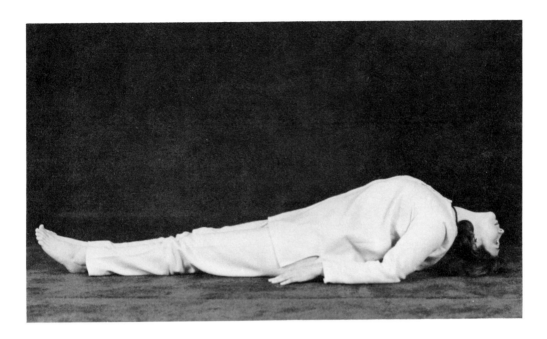

HALF FISH (*Ardha Matsyasana*)

Sit with the head, neck, and trunk straight, legs together and extended in front of the body. Lean back and place the elbows and forearms on the floor, in line with the body and legs. Arch the back, expanding the chest, and stretch the neck backward, placing the crown of the head on the floor. Increase the stretch by further arching the back and pulling the head as far as you can toward the back. Be sure to keep the mouth closed to maintain the stretch in the neck.

Breathe evenly; hold for 15 to 20 seconds.

Gently lower the body to a prone position. Relax.

As one advances, this posture can also be done from a prone position by arching the back and bringing the top of the head to the floor.

Benefits:

- Provides a stretch to the cervical vertebrae complementary to that of the shoulderstand. It amplifies the effects of the shoulderstand and eliminates the slight stiffness in the neck and back that results from doing the shoulderstand alone.

- Expands the chest, promoting deep inhalation, giving good ventilation to the top of the lungs and increasing their capacity.

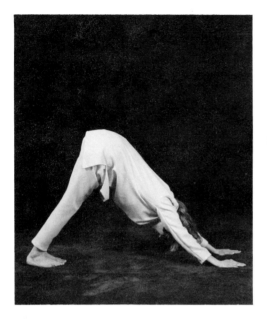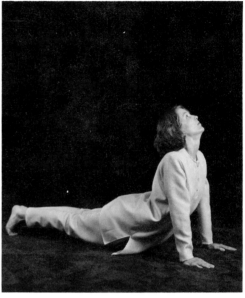

PREPARATION FOR THE HEADSTAND

These two preparatory exercises strengthen the muscles of the arms and shoulders.

EXERCISE 1

Assume position 8 of the sun salutation, as shown above in the left photograph (and described on p. 55).

Exhaling, bend the elbows and bring the head as close to the floor as possible between the hands. The nose and chin should not touch the floor; the heels will rise during the movement.

Inhaling, continue to bring the head forward and up. Arch the back so that only the hands and toes remain on the floor.

Return to the original position by pushing the buttocks upward and bringing the head back down between the arms and hands.

Repeat the exercise two more times.

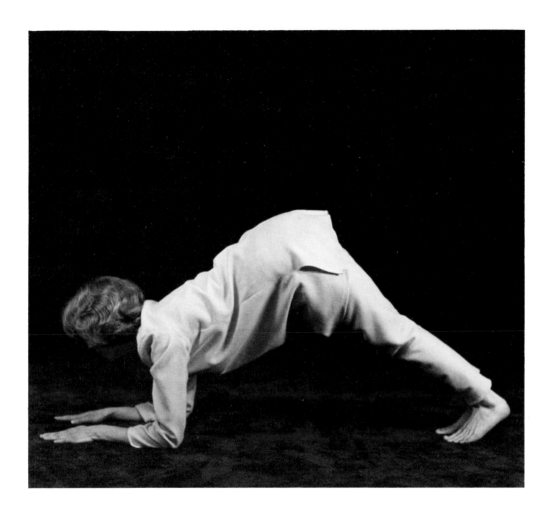

EXERCISE 2

Follow the directions in the first paragraph of step 1 of the headstand (see p. 162).
Then straighten the legs but do *not* walk the feet toward the body.

Keeping the elbows in position, place the hands and forearms on the floor parallel to
each other and pointing away from the head. Raise the head and look up as high as
possible. Hold for 3 seconds. Lower the head, interlace the fingers, and return the
head and knees to the floor; relax.

Repeat two more times.

This posture is sometimes referred to as the dolphin posture.

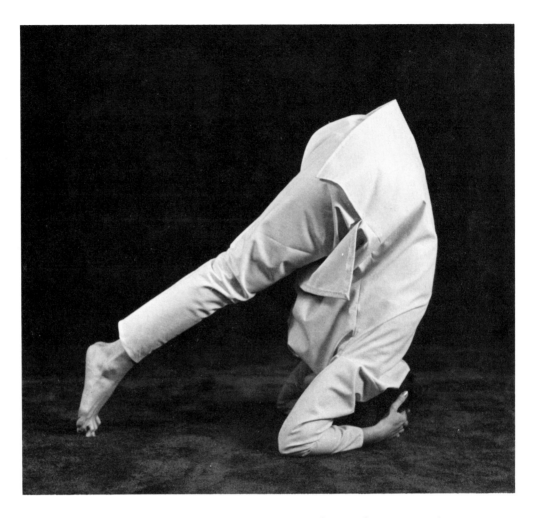

HEADSTAND (*Shirshasana*)

STEP 1

Sit in a kneeling position, interlace the fingers, and place the hands and forearms on the floor approximately 6 to 9 inches in front of the knees. The elbows should be no further than a forearm's width apart. Raise the hips slightly and place the head—specifically, that area approximately 2 inches in front of the crown of the head—on the floor. The interlaced fingers support the back of the head; most of the weight of the body is supported by the hands and forearms.

Straighten the legs and walk the feet toward the body until the hips are over the shoulders and the back is perpendicular to the floor. At this point, more pressure will be felt on the head and neck. However, the arms and hands should still support most of the body's weight so that the head and neck muscles are not strained.

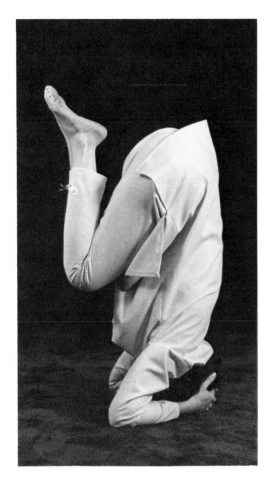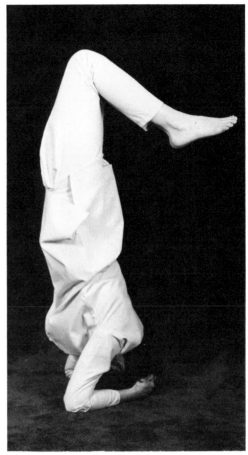

STEP 2

Keeping the back straight, raise both legs, bringing the knees toward the chest and the heels toward the buttocks.

If you find it difficult to raise both legs at the same time and maintain balance, slowly raise one leg while keeping the other on the floor. When this becomes steady, raise the other leg. Do not jerk the legs up suddenly or raise them without complete control. This position is the foundation of the headstand; therefore, it is important that you master it before continuing. Practice this position until you can hold it comfortably for at least 30 seconds before proceeding.

STEP 3

Keeping the heels close to the buttocks, slowly raise the legs until the thighs are perpendicular to the floor. The knees point toward the ceiling and the lower legs are bent loosely behind the upper legs.

STEP 4

Keeping the body stable, slowly raise the lower legs until the feet point toward the ceiling. Breathe evenly. Remember to concentrate most of the body's weight on the elbows and forearms. Hold this position only as long as it is comfortable. If at any time you feel discomfort in the head or neck, come out of the posture. Gradually increase the length of time until you can hold this position for one minute.

STEP 5

Slowly come out of the posture by reversing the sequence of movements, and return to a sitting position. Maintain the same control coming out of the headstand that you practiced while entering it.

STEP 6

After returning to a sitting position, stand up very slowly. Remain standing for as long as you held the posture. This allows the blood flow to return to normal.

STEP 7

Lie in the corpse posture (described on p. 14); relax completely.

Steps 6 and 7 are part of the headstand and are as important as the first 5 steps. You may therefore find it convenient to do the headstand last in your sequence of asanas, as the body at the end of this exercise is in the corpse posture, which is the position assumed for the concluding relaxation exercise.

Cautions: The headstand is a strenuous posture and should be approached with caution. Even young healthy persons should practice hatha yoga daily for two to three months before attempting the headstand. Persons with the following conditions should not practice this asana: high blood pressure, active sinus infection, acute head cold, glaucoma, neck problems, osteoporosis, weakness in the shoulders, obesity, arthritis. Practicing with any of the last five conditions listed may cause the vertebrae to be crushed, resulting in irreversible damage. Persons over fifty-five should exercise extreme caution because studies have shown that as we get older it is much more difficult for the body to absorb and maintain adequate calcium levels in the bones, and thus by age fifty-five a mild degree of osteoporosis may already have begun. The headstand should also not be practiced during menstruation or pregnancy. Do not practice the posture against walls or near furniture or windows.

Benefits:

- Called "the King of Asanas" and considered a panacea for all diseases.
- Increases the flow of blood to the brain and the blood pressure in the brain.
- Brings exhilaration of spirit and fills the body with energy.
- Is said to increase memory and intelligence.

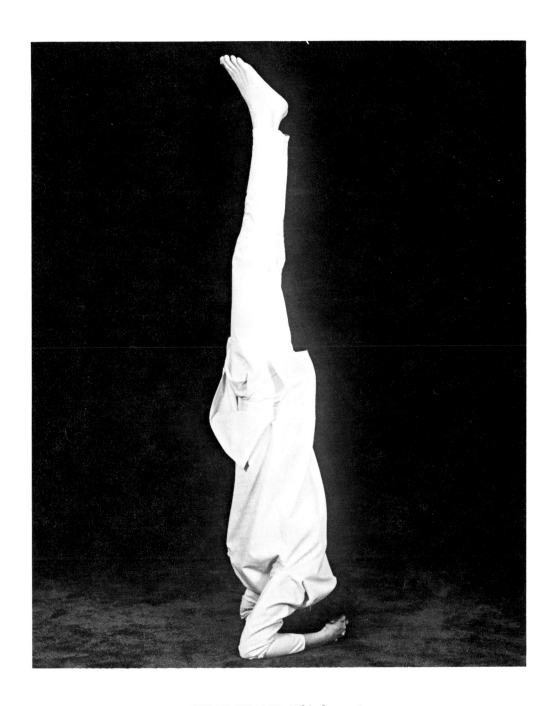

HEADSTAND (*Shirshasana*)

RELAXATION EXERCISES

Tension/Relaxation Exercise

This exercise is done for 3 minutes at the beginning of your hatha yoga session. It can be practiced for several weeks or until the body and mind have started letting go of tension through the practice of hatha yoga postures, breathing exercises, and meditation.

Technique

Lie in the corpse posture (described on p. 14), relaxed and breathing evenly. With the eyes opened wide, open the mouth and stretch the tongue out and down. Then retract the tongue, close the mouth, and relax.

Tense all the muscles of the face, pulling them toward the tip of the nose. Then release the tension and relax.

Gently close the eyes, and keep them closed throughout the rest of the exercise.

Gently roll the head side to side several times.

Pull the shoulders forward. Gently release and relax.

Tense the right arm in a subtle manner without making a fist or lifting the arm off the floor. Do not focus exclusively on tensing just the external muscles; take your mind to deeper within the muscle structure. Then release the tension and relax.

Repeat with the left arm.

Tense the hips and the buttocks. Then release the tension and relax.

Tense the right leg in the same manner that you tensed the right arm. Then release the tension and relax.

Repeat with the left leg.

Starting at the toes, relax the body from the toes, through the legs, torso, arms, neck, and head.

Complete Relaxation Exercise

After the postures it is beneficial to do a concentrated relaxation exercise. There are many such exercises. (For an extensive presentation of such exercises, see *Exercise Without Movement,* a Himalayan Institute publication.) The one described here relaxes the skeletal muscles, eliminates any fatigue or strain following the postures, and energizes both the mind and the body. During this exercise keep the mind alert and concentrated on your breath as you progressively relax your muscles. In the beginning you should practice this exercise for only 10 minutes, because beyond that time the mind usually begins to wander and you may find yourself drifting toward sleep.

Technique

Lie in the corpse posture (described on p. 14) with the eyes gently closed. Inhale and exhale through the nostrils slowly, smoothly, and deeply. There should be no noise, jerks, or pauses in the breath; let the inhalations and exhalations flow naturally without exertion in one continuous movement. Keep the body still.

Mentally travel through the body and relax the top of the head, forehead, eyebrows, space between the eyebrows, eyes, eyelids, cheeks, and nose. Then exhale and inhale completely four times.

Relax the mouth, jaw, chin, neck, shoulders, upper arms, lower arms, wrists, hands, fingers, and fingertips. Feel as if you are exhaling from the fingertips, up the arms, shoulders, and face to the nostrils, and inhaling back to the fingertips. Then exhale and inhale completely four times.

Relax the fingertips, fingers, hands, wrists, lower arms, upper arms, shoulders, upper back, and chest. Concentrate at the center of the chest, and exhale and inhale completely four times.

Relax the stomach, abdomen, lower back, hips, thighs, knees, calves, ankles, feet, and toes. Exhale as though your whole body is exhaling, and inhale as though your whole body is inhaling. Expel all your tension, worries, and anxieties; inhale vital energy, peace, and relaxation. Exhale and inhale completely four times.

Relax the toes, feet, ankles, calves, thighs, knees, hips, lower back, abdomen, stomach, and chest. Concentrating at the center of the chest, exhale and inhale completely four times.

Relax the upper back, shoulders, upper arms, lower arms, wrists, hands, fingers, and fingertips. Then exhale and inhale completely four times.

Relax the fingertips, fingers, hands, wrists, lower arms, upper arms, shoulders, neck, chin, jaw, mouth, and nostrils. Then exhale and inhale completely four times.

Relax the cheeks, eyelids, eyes, eyebrows, space between the eyebrows, forehead, and top of the head. Now, for 30 to 60 seconds, let your mind be aware of the calm and serene flow of the breath; let your mind make a gentle, conscious effort to guide your breath so that it remains smooth, calm, and deep, without any noise or jerks.

Slowly and gently open your eyes. Stretch the body. Try to maintain this calm, peaceful feeling throughout the day.

BREATHING EXERCISES

Pranayama—Control of Breath

Pranayama, the science of breath, follows *asanas* as the fourth rung on the ladder of raja yoga as outlined by Patanjali (see p. 1 of the Introduction). The perfection of yoga asanas leads one to a natural awareness and deeper understanding of breath and its variations. It is necessary to develop this awareness of breath along with the habit of diaphragmatic breathing before beginning the practice of pranayama.

Dividing the word *pranayama* clarifies its meaning. *Prana* means "life force" and *yama* means "control"; thus, pranayama is the control of the life force. Prana, or life force, refers to the total latent and active energies in the human being and the universe. This energy in its many manifestations sustains us; it is the vital energy in the sunlight, in the food we eat, and in the air we breathe. Breath is a vehicle for prana; it carries one of the most subtle forms of this vital energy. Therefore, the first and most important step in the practice of pranayama is learning to regulate the breath, thereby having control over the motion of the lungs.

Active and Passive Nostrils

Usually the breath does not flow equally in both nostrils; one nostril is more congested than the other. This can be easily observed: gently close one nostril and inhale and exhale rapidly through the open nostril; then repeat the process on the opposite side. You will find that one nostril flows more freely than the other; this one is the active nostril, the other is the passive nostril. One inhales prana through the active nostril and exhales prana through the passive nostril. Throughout the day and night the active and passive nostrils alternate. According to yoga science this phenomenon is the result of the alternating flow of subtle energy in *ida* and *pingala,* the two main energy channels (*nadis*) along the spinal column. For meditation, it is desirable to activate these two *nadis* equally and apply *sushumna* (the state of joy in which both nostrils flow freely).

For a thorough presentation of the science of breath, see *Science of Breath: A Practical Guide* by Swami Rama, Rudolph Ballentine, M.D., and Alan Hymes, M.D. (a Himalayan Institute publication).

172

The Complete Breath

The complete breath helps expand the capacity of the lungs and is excellent as a physically and mentally energizing exercise. If possible, practice the exercise in front of an open window or out of doors.

When doing the exercise it may be helpful to imagine yourself as a glass of water being emptied and filled. When the water is poured out, the glass empties from the top to the bottom. When the water is poured in, the glass fills from the bottom to the top.

Technique

Assume the simple standing posture.

Inhaling, fill the lower lungs, then the middle lungs, and then the upper lungs; simultaneously, raise the arms until they are overhead, palms touching, in a prayer position.

Exhaling, empty the upper lungs, then the middle lungs, and then the lower lungs as the arms are lowered back to the sides.

Repeat the exercise 2 to 5 more times.

Nadi Shodhana

There are many methods of pranayama, each for a specific purpose. *Nadi shodhana* is a simple pranayama exercise that purifies the *nadis,* the subtle energy channels. It balances the flow of breath in the nostrils and the flow of energy in the nadis. Nadi shodhana should be practiced at least twice a day, in the morning and evening.

A. Sit in the easy posture (see p. 88) with the head, neck, and trunk straight. Inhalation and exhalation should be of equal duration. Do not force the breath; keep it slow, controlled, and free from sounds and jerks. With practice, gradually lengthen the duration of the inhalation and the exhalation.

B. Bring the right hand to the nose, folding the index finger and the middle finger so that the right thumb can be used to close the right nostril and the ring finger can be used to close the left nostril.

C. Close the passive nostril and exhale completely through the active nostril.

D. At the end of the exhalation, close the active nostril and inhale through the passive nostril slowly and completely. Inhalation and exhalation should be of equal duration.

E. Repeat this cycle of exhalation with the active nostril and inhalation with the passive nostril two more times.

F. At the end of the third inhalation with the passive nostril, exhale completely through the same nostril, keeping the active nostril closed with the finger or thumb.

G. At the end of the exhalation, close the passive nostril and inhale through the active nostril.

H. Repeat two more times the cycle of exhalation through the passive nostril and inhalation through the active nostril.

I. To sum up:

1	Exhale	Active
2	Inhale	Passive
3	Exhale	Active
4	Inhale	Passive
5	Exhale	Active
6	Inhale	Passive
7	Exhale	Passive
8	Inhale	Active
9	Exhale	Passive
10	Inhale	Active
11	Exhale	Passive
12	Inhale	Active

J. Place the hands on the knees and exhale and inhale through both nostrils evenly for three complete breaths. This completes ONE cycle of nadi shodhana.

Kapalabhati Pranayama

Once diaphragmatic breathing has become a natural, unconscious function and nadi shodhana has been practiced for two to three months, then kapalabhati may be practiced.

Literally, *kapalabhati* means the pranayama that "makes the skull shine." Sit with the head, neck, and trunk in a straight line. Using the diaphragm and the abdominal muscles, quickly and forcefully expel the breath. This is followed by a slow, spontaneous inhalation as the abdominal muscles are relaxed. This constitutes one cycle; the cycles are repeated in rapid succession. Begin with seven cycles and slowly increase to twenty-one. This exercise cleans the sinuses and respiratory passages and stimulates the digestive organs.

Appendix A

Sample Lesson Plans

At the Himalayan Institute, beginning I and II hatha yoga classes meet for eight weeks, one and a half hours per class. In the first few weeks of practice, students are encouraged to focus on the joints and glands exercises, on the stretching exercises, and on proper breathing and relaxation techniques. Gradually, new postures are added to the practice.

Following are 30-minute, 60-minute, and 90-minute sample lesson plans for the beginning I and beginning II levels. These lessons are intended for students in their first few weeks of practice at each level. Gradually, according to individual capacity, new postures and variations may be added.

BEGINNING I: 30 Minutes

Centering:	Tension/Relaxation
Limbering:	Forehead and Sinus Massage* Neck Rolls* Cat Stretch
Standing:	Simple Standing Posture Shoulder Rotations* Horizontal Arm Swing* Overhead Stretch Side Stretch Simple Back Stretch Leg Kicks* Ankles and Feet*
Sitting:	Leg Cradles
Backward-Bending:	Cobra
Forward-Bending:	Child's Posture
Twisting:	Twisting Posture
Leg Lifts:	Knees-to-Chest Posture
Relaxation:	Complete Relaxation (3 to 5 minutes)

*Not described in this manual. For a description of this exercise, see the Himalayan Institute publication *Joints and Glands Exercises.*

176

BEGINNING I: 60 Minutes

Centering:	Tension/Relaxation
	Symmetrical Stretch
Limbering:	Forehead and Sinus Massage*
	Eye Exercises*
	Neck Rolls*
	Cat Stretch
Standing:	Simple Standing Posture
	Shoulder Rotations*
	Horizontal Arm Swing*
	Overhead Stretch
	Side Stretch
	Torso Twist
	Leg Kicks*
	Ankles and Feet*
Sitting:	Leg Cradles
	Rocking Chair
Backward-Bending:	Cobra
	Half Locust
Forward-Bending:	Child's Posture
	Churning
Twisting:	Twisting Posture
Leg Lifts:	Knees-to-Chest Posture
	Wind-Eliminating Posture
Inverted:	Arch Posture
Relaxation:	Complete Relaxation (5 minutes)

*Not described in this manual. For a description of this exercise, see the Himalayan Institute publication *Joints and Glands Exercises.*

BEGINNING I: 90 Minutes

Centering: Breath Awareness in Corpse Posture
                         Symmetrical Stretch

Limbering: Forehead and Sinus Massage*
                         Scalp and Forehead*
                         Eye Exercises*
                         Mouth Exercise*
                         Face Massage*
                         Neck Rolls*
                         Cat Stretch

Standing: Simple Standing Posture
                         Shoulder Lifts*
                         Shoulder Rotations*
                         Horizontal Arm Swing*
                         Arms, Hands, and Wrists*
                         Relaxation in Corpse Posture (1 to 2 minutes)
                         Horizontal Stretch
                         Overhead Stretch
                         Side Stretch
                         Simple Back Stretch
                         Torso Twist
                         Leg Kicks*
                         Knee Swirls*
                         Ankles and Feet*

Sitting: Leg Cradles
                         Rocking Chair

Backward-Bending: Cobra
                         Crocodile
                         Half Locust
                         Half Bow

Forward-Bending: Child's Posture
                         Churning

Twisting: Twisting Posture

Leg Lifts: Knees-to-Chest Posture
                         Wind-Eliminating Posture

Inverted: Arch Posture

Relaxation: Complete Relaxation (5 to 10 minutes)

*Not described in this manual. For a description of this exercise, see the Himalayan Institute publication *Joints and Glands Exercises.*

178

BEGINNING II: 30 Minutes

Centering: Diaphragmatic Breathing in Corpse Posture
                        Uddiyana Bandha

Limbering: Sun Salutation (2 to 3 times)

Standing: Overhead Stretch
                        Side Stretch
                        Triangle
                        Tree

Sitting: Squatting Posture
                        Leg Cradles

Backward-Bending: Cobra
                        Crocodile
                        Locust
                        Half Bow

Forward-Bending: Child's Posture
                        Butterfly
                        Head-to-Knee Posture

Twisting: Half Spinal Twist

Inverted: Half Plow
                        Inverted Action Posture
                        Half Fish

Relaxation: Complete Relaxation (5 minutes)

BEGINNING II: 60 Minutes

Centering: Diaphragmatic Breathing in Corpse Posture
Uddiyana Bandha

Limbering: Neck Rolls*
Sun Salutation (3 times)

Standing: Side Stretch
Triangle
Preparation for Revolving Triangle
Tree
Hand-to-Foot Posture

Sitting: Squatting Posture
Leg Cradles

Backward-Bending: Horse Mudra in Crocodile Posture
Cobra
Crocodile
Locust
Half Bow

Forward-Bending: Child's Posture
Butterfly
Head-to-Knee Posture

Twisting: Half Spinal Twist

Leg Lifts: Single Leg Lifts

Inverted: Half Plow
Inverted Action Posture
Arch Posture
Half Fish

Relaxation: Complete Relaxation (5 minutes)

Breathing: Nadi Shodhana

*Not described in this manual. For a description of this exercise, see the Himalayan Institute publication *Joints and Glands Exercises.*

BEGINNING II: 90 Minutes

Centering: Diaphragmatic Breathing in Corpse Posture
Easy Posture
Uddiyana Bandha

Limbering: Neck Rolls*
Sun Salutation (3 times)

Standing: Overhead Stretch
Side Bend
Angle Posture
Triangle
Preparation for Revolving Triangle
Tree
Hand-to-Foot Posture

Sitting: Squatting Posture
Leg Cradles
Half Lotus
Yoga Mudra in Easy Posture

Backward-Bending: Horse Mudra in Crocodile Posture
Cobra
Crocodile
Locust
Half Bow

Forward-Bending: Child's Posture
Butterfly
Head-to-Knee Posture
Posterior Stretch

Twisting: Half Spinal Twist

Leg Lifts: Single Leg Lifts
Double Leg Lifts

Inverted: Half Plow
Inverted Action Posture
Arch Posture
Half Fish

Relaxation: Complete Relaxation (10 minutes)

Breathing: Nadi Shodhana

*Not described in this manual. For a description of this exercise, see the Himalayan Institute publication *Joints and Glands Exercises*.

Appendix B

Hatha Yoga and Menstruation
by Barbara Bova

It is generally not recommended to do postures during the menstrual period, particularly not during the initial days when the flow is the heaviest. Rather it is advisable to relax as much as possible during the menses and to refrain from physical exercise for at least three days. This advice may seem surprising, since the modern attitude has become such that we are encouraged to ignore the menstrual period and to make no adjustments in our regular routine to accommodate it. However, practicing postures or engaging in other strenuous exercise at this time may increase cramps or cause excessive bleeding.

Menstruation is a highly complex process, set in motion and maintained by a very subtle and delicate mechanism that is dependent not only on physiological homeostasis but also on energetic, emotional, and mental equilibrium. The slightest upset of the state of balance can result in menstrual irregularities and disorders. Because the cause of these disturbances may be so subtle that it is not possible to be detected by modern scientific diagnostic techniques, it may take months, or even years, to reestablish the equilibrium for the reproductive system to regain its natural state of order and efficiency.

Unfortunately, popular use of the birth control pill has reduced the menstrual cycle to a mechanical process, externally initiated and controlled, with little or no awareness on the part of the individual woman. It is important to develop self-awareness and sensitivity to what is happening within the body because the more aware we are of the subtleties of the body when it is functioning normally, the more likely we are to notice slight changes that could indicate the initial stages of disease. If we are able to detect a potential problem from the start, we can prevent it from deteriorating into a serious or permanent disorder. In addition, awareness engenders self-reliance, allowing us to be responsible for the health of our own bodies and eliminating dependency on intrusive modalities such as drugs or surgery, which may in themselves create additional problems.

Hatha yoga is a means of regaining or developing body awareness, of getting back in touch with the body's signals and needs. A consistent practice of hatha yoga during the rest of the month can be beneficial for either maintaining or reestablishing order in the process of menstruation. The longer you practice hatha, the more sensitive you will become to the subtle changes that take place in the body in preparation for menstruation.

For example, a couple of days before the menstrual period begins you may notice that the body is less willing to do postures, and may feel less flexible or even sluggish. This is a message from the body indicating that it is time to slow down and take it easy. Do not misinterpret this message to mean that you are becoming lazy and mistakenly try to force your body to perform, as this can result in injury. You may also have the tendency to think it is your imagination or a coincidence that you have less energy immediately prior to the commencement of the menses. The concept of prana (life force) as explained by yoga science and philosophy is helpful in understanding why this energy lag occurs.

According to yoga science there are many different types of prana that are responsible for the functioning of the biological processes within the body. The five of these which are most important and their respective responsibilities are: *prana* (absorption, respiration); *apana* (elimination, excretory system); *samana* (assimilation, digestive system); *vyana* (circulation); and *udana* (expression). Apana is the energy responsible for downward-flowing movement, and it is this downward motion of apana that initiates the monthly cleansing process in the uterus. Because in the performance of postures the energy is being directed in many different directions, doing postures during the menstrual period confuses the body and interrupts this natural tendency of the downward and outward cleansing movement.

This is why it is especially advised not to do any inverted postures or uddiyana bandha, agnisara, and nauli, as these all act to redirect the apana energy upward. It is because of the concentration of energy that is moving down and out that the rest of the body feels less energetic at this time. This is natural and should not be resisted or ignored. It is important simply to be aware of the changes taking place and to observe them.

If you feel that you need to do something to help relieve cramps and to make yourself feel more comfortable, the simple squatting posture may be helpful, and practicing diaphragmatic breathing and doing a systematic relaxation lying in the corpse pose are also beneficial. Practicing smooth, deep, even, diaphragmatic breathing and mentally observing the rhythmic flow of inhalation and exhalation helps to create a state of calmness.

The important thing is to remember that you are an individual and that your needs are unique to you. It is your responsibility to become sensitive to what those needs are and then to supply them according to your capacity. The menses may be thought of as a special opportunity to apply more time to spiritual readings and meditative practices and to experience more fully the natural female aspect of being in touch with the flow of nature.

Reprinted, by permission, from *Dawn* magazine (vol. 3, no. 1), a Himalayan Institute publication.

About the Authors

Samskrti (Linda Blanchard) received a B.A. in Religious Studies from the University of Minnesota. She has studied and practiced hatha and raja yoga since 1971 and received training at Shri Swami Rama's ashram, Rishikesh, India, as well as at the Himalayan Institute's American headquarters. She has taught hatha yoga since 1972.

Veda (Rosalie Currey) has been studying hatha and raja yoga under the guidance of Shri Swami Rama since 1972, including a two-year residential program at the Himalayan Institute's national headquarters. She has also traveled to India for further study of yoga. She has taught hatha yoga since 1973.

The Himalayan Institute Teachers' Association and Diploma Program

The Himalayan Institute Diploma Program offers students a systematic study and practice of raja yoga. Beginning with hatha yoga and the development of stamina, flexibility, and control of the body, the courses proceed through the practice of meditation to concentration of attention and expansion of awareness. Through this ancient method, also called ashtanga or eight-limbed yoga, the mind and breath become steady and actions are performed skillfully.

Students may join this ongoing program at any time and begin taking the required classes as they are offered. For those students who are seriously considering taking the major step of becoming a yoga teacher, certification in the Himalayan Institute Teachers' Association (HITA) is available upon completion of the Intermediate level of the Diploma Program. The primary goal of HITA is to conduct, under the spiritual guidance and in the tradition of Shri Swami Rama, a professional organization of teachers of yoga with standardized criteria of competency.

Course requirements for the Diploma Program include the following:

Beginning Level—Beginning Hatha Yoga I and II, Introduction to Meditation, Diet and Nutrition, and two reports, one on a diet and nutrition experiment and one on personal meditation practice.

Intermediate Level—Intermediate Hatha Yoga I and II, Science of Breath, Superconscious Meditation I, Yoga Sutras, Yoga Anatomy, examination and board appearance for teacher's certification if desired.

Advanced level—Advanced Hatha Yoga, Advanced Yoga Anatomy, Hatha-yogapradipika, Yoga Sutras II, Superconscious Meditation II, plus an elective from one of the following:

    a. Bhagavad Gita

    b. Upanishads

    c. Sankhya Philosophy

Written and oral examinations are also taken at the end of the advanced-level study program.

Completion of the intermediate-level Diploma Program courses along with a written and oral examination are prerequisites for teacher's certification and membership in HITA.

For further information on the Diploma Program or HITA, or to apply to the Diploma Program, please write to the Himalayan Institute, 1505 Greenwood Road, Glenview, IL 60025.

For information on the residential study program, please write to the Himalayan Institute Residential Program, RR 1, Box 400, Honesdale, PA 18431.

Index

Abdominal lift (*uddiyana bandha*), 66
Adho mukha shvanasana (dog-stretch), 45
Angle posture (*konasana*), 68-71
Arch posture, 158
Ardha dhanurasana (half bow), 120
Ardha halasana (half plow), 150
Ardha matsyasana (half fish), 159
Ardha matsyendrasana (half spinal twist), 136
Ardha naukasana (half boat), 114
Ardha padmasana (half lotus), 90
Ardha shalabhasana (half locust), 118
Ashtanga yoga, 1
Ashvini mudra (horse mudra), 112

Back-bending posture (*urdhvasana*), 45
Back stretch, simple, 34
Balance on hips (*utthita hastapadasana*), 144
Balasana (child's posture), 18
Bhujangasana (cobra), 110
Boat (*naukasana*), 116. *See also* Balance on
  hips
  half, 114
Bow (*dhanurasana*), 122
  half, 120
Breathing
  diaphragmatic, 10-12
  exercises, 171-74
Butterfly, 96

Cat stretch, 26
Chalan (churning), 40
Child's posture (*balasana*), 18
Churning (*chalan*), 40
Cobra (*bhujangasana*), 110
Complete breath, 173
Corpse (*shavasana*), 14
Cow's face (*gomukhasana*), 104-7
Cradles, leg, 92-95
Crocodile (*makarasana*), 16

Dhanurasana (bow), 122
  half bow, 120
Dog-stretch (*adho mukha shvanasana*), 45
Dolphin, 161
Double leg lifts (*utthita dvipadasana*), 143

Easy posture (*sukhasana*), 88

Fish, half (*ardha matsyasana*), 159

Gomukasana (cow's face), 104-7

Halasana (plow), 152
  half plow, 150
Half spinal twist (*ardha matsyendrasana*), 136
Hand-to-foot posture (*padahastasana*), 84
  preparation for, 82
Hathayogapradipika (Svatmarama), 2
Headstand (*shirshasana*), 162-65
  preparation for, 160
Head-to-knee posture (*janushirshasana*), 126
  preparation for, 125
Horizontal stretch, 28
Horse mudra (*ashvini mudra*), 112

Inclined plane (*katikasana*), 130
Inverted action posture (*vipritakarani*), 154

Janushirshasana (head-to-knee posture), 126
  preparation for, 125
Joints and Glands Exercises (ed. Ballentine), 3

Kapalabhati pranayama, 174
Katikasana (inclined plane), 130
"King of Asanas," 164
Kneeling posture (*vajrasana*), 89
Knees-to-chest posture, 20
Konasana (angle posture), 68-71

Lectures on Yoga (Rama), 3
Leg cradles, 92-95
Leg lifts
  double (*utthita dvipadasana*), 143
  single (*utthita ekapadasana*), 140
Lion (*simhasana*), 98
Locust (*shalabhasana*), 119
  half, 118
Lotus, half (*ardha padmasana*), 90

Makarasana (crocodile), 16
Menstruation, 182-83

Nadi shodhana, 173-74
Naukasana (boat), 116
  half boat, 114
Niyamas, 8-9
Nostrils, active and passive, 172

Overhead stretch, 30

Padahastasana (hand-to-foot posture), 84
        preparation for, 82
Parivritta trikonasana (revolving triangle), 76
        preparation for, 74
Paschimottanasana (posterior stretch), 128
        preparation for, 125
Patanjali, 1-2
Pavanamuktasana (wind-eliminating posture),
        139
Plow (*halasana*), 152
        half, 150
Posterior stretch (*paschimottanasana*), 128
        preparation for, 125
Pranayama, 172-74

"Queen of Asanas," 156

Raja yoga, 1
Relaxation
        exercises, 167-70
        postures, 13-21
Revolving triangle (*parivritta trikonasana*), 76
        preparation for, 74
Rocking chair, 148

Salutation, sun (*surya namaskara*), 43-59
Sarvangasana (shoulderstand), 156
Shalabhasana (locust), 119
        half locust, 118
Shavasana (corpse), 14
Shirshasana (headstand), 162-65
        preparation for, 160
Shoulderstand (*sarvangasana*), 156
Side stretch, 32
Simhasana (lion), 98
Simple back stretch, 34
Simple standing posture, 21
Single leg lifts (*utthita ekapadasana*), 140
Spinal twist, half (*ardha matsyendrasana*),
        136
Squatting posture, 102
Standing posture, simple, 21
Stretch
        back, 34
        cat, 26
        horizontal, 28
        overhead, 30
        side, 32
        swimming, 38
Sukhasana (easy posture), 88
Sun salutation (*surya namaskara*), 43-59
Surya namaskara (sun salutation), 43-59
Svatmarama, 2
Swimming stretch, 38
Symbol of yoga (*yoga mudra*), 100
Symmetrical stretch, 24

Torso twist, 36
Tree (*vrikshasana*), 78-81
Triangle (*trikonasana*), 72
        revolving, 76
                preparation for, 74

Trikonasana (triangle), 72
        revolving triangle, 76
                preparation for, 74
Twist, torso, 36
Twisting posture, 134

Uddiyana bandha (abdominal lift), 66
Urdhvasana (back-bending posture), 45
Utthita dvipadasana (double leg lifts), 143
Utthita ekapadasana (single leg lifts), 140
Utthita hastapadasana (balance on hips), 144

Vajrasana (kneeling posture), 89
Vipritakarani (inverted action posture), 154
Vrikshasana (tree), 78-81

Wind-eliminating posture
                (*pavanamuktasana*), 139

Yamas, 8
Yoga mudra (symbol of yoga), 100
Yoga Sutras, 1-2

Zen posture (*vajrasana*), 89

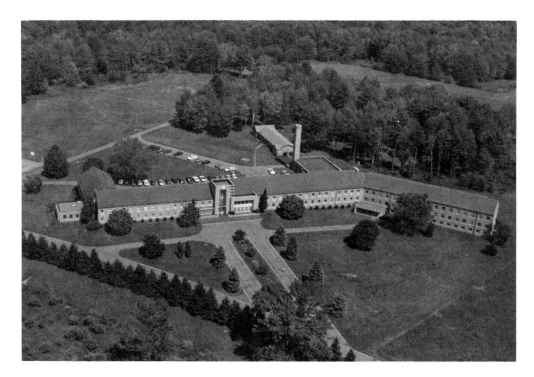

The main building of the national headquarters, Honesdale, Pa.

The Himalayan Institute

The Himalayan International Institute of Yoga Science and Philosophy of the U.S.A. is a nonprofit organization devoted to the scientific and spiritual progress of modern humanity. Founded in 1971 by Sri Swami Rama, the Institute combines Western and Eastern teachings and techniques to develop educational, therapeutic, and research programs for serving people in today's world. The goals of the Institute are to teach meditational techniques for the growth of individuals and their society, to make known the harmonious view of world religions and philosophies, and to undertake scientific research for the benefit of humankind.

This challenging task is met by people of all ages, all walks of life, and all faiths who attend and participate in the Institute courses and seminars. These programs, which are given on a continuing basis, are designed in order that one may discover for oneself how to live more creatively. In the words of Swami Rama, "By being aware of one's own potential and abilities, one can become a perfect citizen, help the nation, and serve humanity."

The Institute has branch centers and affiliates throughout the United States. The 422-acre campus of the national headquarters, located in the Pocono Mountains of northeastern Pennsylvania, serves as the coordination center for all the Institute activities, which include a wide variety of innovative programs in education, research, and therapy, combining Eastern and Western approaches to self-awareness and self-directed change.

SEMINARS, LECTURES, WORKSHOPS, and CLASSES are available throughout the year, providing intensive training and experience in such topics as Superconscious Meditation, hatha yoga, philosophy, psychology, and various aspects of personal growth and holistic health. The *Himalayan News,* a free bimonthly publication, announces the current programs.

The RESIDENTIAL and SELF-TRANSFORMATION PROGRAMS provide training in the basic yoga disciplines—diet, ethical behavior, hatha yoga, and meditation.

Students are also given guidance in a philosophy of living in a community environment.

The PROGRAM IN EASTERN STUDIES AND COMPARATIVE PSYCHOL-OGY offers a unique and systematic synthesis of Western empirical sources and Eastern introspective science. Masters and Doctoral-level studies may be pursued through cross-registration with several accredited colleges and universities.

The five-day STRESS MANAGEMENT/ PHYSICAL FITNESS PROGRAM offers practical and individualized training that can be used to control the stress response. This includes biofeedback, relaxation skills, exercise, diet, breathing techniques, and meditation.

A yearly INTERNATIONAL CONGRESS, sponsored by the Institute, is devoted to the scientific and spiritual progress of modern humanity. Through lectures, workshops, seminars, and practical demonstrations, it provides a forum for professionals and lay people to share their knowledge and research.

The ELEANOR N. DANA RESEARCH LABORATORY is the psychophysiological laboratory of the Institute, specializing in research on breathing, meditation, holistic therapies, and stress and relaxed states. The laboratory is fully equipped for exercise stress testing and psychophysiological measurements, including brain waves, patterns of respiration, heart rate changes, and muscle tension. The staff investigates Eastern teachings through studies based on Western experimental techniques.

Himalayan Institute Publications

Living with the Himalayan Masters	Swami Rama
Lectures on Yoga	Swami Rama
A Practical Guide to Holistic Health	Swami Rama
Choosing a Path	Swami Rama
Inspired Thoughts of Swami Rama	Swami Rama
Freedom from the Bondage of Karma	Swami Rama
Book of Wisdom (Ishopanishad)	Swami Rama
Enlightenment Without God	Swami Rama
Exercise Without Movement	Swami Rama
Life Here and Hereafter	Swami Rama
Marriage, Parenthood, and Enlightenment	Swami Rama
Path of Fire and Light	Swami Rama
Perennial Psychology of the Bhagavad Gita	Swami Rama
Creative Use of Emotion	Swami Rama, Swami Ajaya
Science of Breath	Swami Rama, Rudolph Ballentine, M.D., Alan Hymes, M.D.
Yoga and Psychotherapy	Swami Rama, Rudolph Ballentine, M.D., Swami Ajaya
Superconscious Meditation	Usharbudh Arya, D.Litt.
Mantra and Meditation	Usharbudh Arya, D.Litt.
Philosophy of Hatha Yoga	Usharbudh Arya, D.Litt.
Meditation and the Art of Dying	Usharbudh Arya, D.Litt.
God	Usharbudh Arya, D.Litt.
Yoga-sūtras of Patañjali, Volume I	Usharbudh Arya, D.Litt.
Psychotherapy East and West: A Unifying Paradigm	Swami Ajaya, Ph.D.
Yoga Psychology	Swami Ajaya, Ph.D.
Psychology East and West	Swami Ajaya, Ph.D. (ed.)
Meditational Therapy	Swami Ajaya, Ph.D. (ed.)
Diet and Nutrition	Rudolph Ballentine, M.D.
Joints and Glands Exercises	Rudolph Ballentine, M.D. (ed.)
Theory and Practice of Meditation	Rudolph Ballentine, M.D. (ed.)
Freedom from Stress	Phil Nuernberger, Ph.D.
Science Studies Yoga	James Funderburk, Ph.D.
Homeopathic Remedies	Drs. Anderson, Buegel, Chernin
Hatha Yoga Manual I	Samskrti and Veda
Hatha Yoga Manual II	Samskrti and Judith Franks
Seven Systems of Indian Philosophy	R. Tigunait, Ph.D.
Swami Rama of the Himalayas	L. K. Misra, Ph.D. (ed.)
Philosophy of Death and Dying	M. V. Kamath
Practical Vedanta of Swami Rama Tirtha	Brandt Dayton (ed.)
The Swami and Sam	Brandt Dayton
Yoga Psychology and the Beatitudes	S. Arpita, Ph.D.
Yoga and Christianity	Justin O'Brien, D.Th.
Himalayan Mountain Cookery	Martha Ballentine

The Yoga Way Cookbook	Himalayan Institute
Meditation in Christianity	Himalayan Institute
Art and Science of Meditation	Himalayan institute
Therapeutic Value of Yoga	Himalayan Institute
Chants from Eternity	Himalayan Institute
Spiritual Diary	Himalayan Institute
Blank Books	Himalayan Institute

Write for a free mail order catalog describing all our publications.